*The Right
to Treatment
For Mental Patients*

THE RIGHT
TO TREATMENT
FOR MENTAL PATIENTS

Edited by
STUART GOLANN
and WILLIAM J. FREMOUW

IRVINGTON PUBLISHERS, Inc., New York

Distributed by HALSTED PRESS, Division of

JOHN WILEY & SONS

New York   London   Toronto   Sydney

Distributed by HALSTED PRESS
A division of JOHN WILEY & SONS, New York

Library of Congress Cataloging in Publication Data
Main entry under title:

The right to treatment for mental patients.

    1. Mental health laws—United States—Addresses, essays, lectures. 2. Insanity—Jurisprudence—
United States—Addresses, essays, lectures.
I. Golann, Stuart E.   II. Fremouw, William J.
[DNLM: 1. Mental disorders—Therapy—Congresses.
2. Human rights—Congresses.   WM400 A515r]
KF3828.A75R5   344′.73′044   76-18917
ISBN 0-470-15172-2 (Halsted)

The Amherst Conference on the Right to Treatment was held on May 21-22, 1973. Though the papers in this book are those presented at the Conference, they have been updated to include material that has surfaced up to the time of this publication.

The chapter "A New Right to Treatment," first appeared in *The Journal of Psychiatry and Law* © 1974 and is reprinted with permission of the publisher, Federal Legal Publications, Inc.

The chapter "The Right to Treatment: Judicial Action and Social Change," first appeared in *Politics, Medicine and Social Science* © 1974 and is reprinted with permission of the publisher, John Wiley & Sons, Inc.

Printed in The United States of America

Contents

Contents

Editors' Note

A word of explanation concerning legal references to court cases. These are presented in the standard legal form, that is: *Millard v. Cameron*, 373 F.2d 468 (D.C. Cir. 1966) *Case title:* Millard v. Cameron; *Volume and name (abbreviated) of reporter in which the case appears:* volume 373 of Federal Reporter, second series; *Page number:* 468; *Court:* Circuit Court for the District of Columbia; *Date:* 1966.

Court cases not summarized in legal reporters are cited: *Wyatt v. Stickney,* C. A. 3195-N (M.D. Ala.), Order and Decree of April 13, 1972 at 4. *Case title:* Wyatt v. Stickney; *Case number:* Civil Action No. 3195-N; *Court:* Federal District Court, Middle District for Alabama; *Document:* Order and Decree of April 13, 1972; *Page:* 4.

CONTRIBUTORS

BERTRAM BROWN
Director,
National Institute of Mental Health,
Rockville, Md.

WILLIAM J. FREMOUW
Assistant Professor of Psychology,
West Virginia University,
Morgantown, West Va.

STUART GOLANN
Professor of Psychology,
University of Massachusetts,
Amherst, Mass.

CHARLES HALPERN
Attorney,
Center for Law and Social Policy,
Washington, D.C.

RICHARD T. LOUTTIT
Professor of Psychology,
Head, Department of Psychology,
University of Massachusetts,
Amherst, Mass.

DAVID MECHANIC
Professor of Sociology,
University of Wisconsin,
Madison, Wis.

STONEWALL B. STICKNEY
Former Commissioner,
Alabama Department of Mental Health,
Montgomery, Ala.

Foreword

BERTRAM BROWN

The recent series of right-to-treatment cases has captured the imagination of concerned Americans who deplore the conditions that prevail in many large mental institutions. Simply to search out and publicize such conditions, and rouse public indignation, has been an immense contribution for which the mentally disabled, mental health professionals, and the public can be grateful. But the light turned on the dark corners of the back wards also illuminated a whole new set of issues that are neither morally clearcut nor easy to resolve.

The *Wyatt v. Stickney* decision, mandating vast improvements in state mental institutions to implement the right to treatment, quickly raised a series of vital, pragmatic issues: Where were the new human and material resources to come from? Who would pay for them? Should limited resources go to the large hospitals at the expense of community treatment? No answers have yet been found, and those questions have become key points in the ongoing debate over "rhetoric versus reality." It is to the credit of those who uncovered the problems that they have not attempted to hide from them behind a facade of legal principle. And the debate has been invaluable in raising the consciousness of legislators and the public about the real needs of the mentally disabled.

Along with the practical resource questions, those pressing for the right to treatment have uncovered philosophical problems that have even wider ramifications. How is the legal and moral imperative of the right to adequate treatment to be reconciled with the legal and moral imperative of individual dignity and autonomy—the "right to refuse treatment"? When, if ever, should society be able to determine that an individual's right to make judgments about himself can be overridden by his (socially enforced) right to treatment? And the ethical and resource issues fuse in a basic social concern, the ethics of resource allocation. What level of human need will taxpayers and their representatives find tolerable when weighed against other public priorities?

Again, there are no easy answers. At first the right to treatment seemed so simple, so just, so black and white. But like all really basic human principles, its implications were complex indeed. And when we look at those implications in the harsh light of reality, the issues raised by the right to treatment appear as a dazzling array of grays.

I have found this same phenomenon in the case of pretrial diversion from the criminal justice system, where the right to a full trial must be weighed against the chance for meaningful rehabilitation. And, I have recently experienced just how confusing the right-to-treatment issue itself can be. When an impressive group of professional organizations, in many of which I am an active member or officer, sued me (along with the District of Columbia, Saint Elizabeths Hospital, and HEW) to establish a "right to the least restrictive alternative" treatment, the conflict became classically internalized: My professional self was suing my political self.

Even if we could resolve the underlying practical and philosophical dilemmas, we come right back to another question that Judge Johnson grappled with in *Wyatt*. What is "adequate treatment"? In responding to that question society looks to the mental health field for expert guidance. And we must face the sobering question, what is it that we can really offer to those suffering from mental disability?

As the Amherst conference, and the authors of these papers, clearly recognized, the idea of a right to treatment has raised the most fundamental questions about mental health care in our society. It is a tribute to the sincerity, ability, and intellectual honesty of those who have led the movement, that before the "right to treatment" has even been established as a principle of law, they have begun to confront the deeply discomfiting issues that lie at its heart.

Introduction

The Amherst Conference on Right to Treatment was a most timely effort to focus the attention and concern of scholars and practitioners from a variety of disciplines: law, psychology, psychiatry, legal medicine, economics, sociology, etc., on the problems of right to treatment, especially as they have been reflected recently in class action suits. This resulting volume will be a major and valuable contribution to the growing discussion over the rights of institutionalized persons and the problems of implementing these newly restated rights.

All of the professional societies having an interest in the issues to which the conference was addressed were invited to send representatives. While not all did so, it is the organizers hope that the participating organizations will use the conference results in their own efforts to improve the care and treatment offered to the mentally ill and mentally retarded citizens who are in their charge. This volume should provide further assistance to all mental health professionals toward this end.

In welcoming the participants to the conference, I closed my remarks by quoting attorney Charles Halpern:

Perhaps the most alarming potential result of the recent litigation would be if nothing happens; and it must be stressed that that is a very distinct possibility. Too often we have seen important legal principles stated and found that they have had little impact on the real world. Civil rights lawyers, welfare reform lawyers and poverty lawyers have learned a lesson in recent years that people concerned with the mentally retarded have long known: transitory victories and paroxysms of righteous indignation do not change institutions.

In the opening chapter, William Fremouw provides the historical background for and notes the legal evolution of the right-to-treatment concept. He notes the difficulty and complexity of creating standards of treatment and the extensive problems of enforcement of any standards at all.

Stonewall Stickney, in "The Right to Treatment in Alabama," provides a very enlightening insight into the problems of providing proper mental health care in a state without adequate resources or interest. As a defendant in *Wyatt v. Stickney,* he attempted to focus on flexibility and experimentation in offering treatment to mental hospital patients. He also stressed the evaluation of treatment programs through outcome measures rather than through inputs such as number of staff or physical facilities. The serious possibility that court decisions in right-to-treatment cases might inhibit advances and innovations in treatment methods is brought into focus at the end of his chapter.

Sociologist David Mechanic uses the *Wyatt v. Stickney* case as a basis for a broader consideration of the role of courts in bringing about social change. He stresses the continuing discrepancy between judicial edicts and the realities of resources. He further notes that "the right-to-treatment issue alerts us to a fundamental difficulty—the failure to insure an adequate level of treatment entitlement to citizens as a whole."

Attorney Charles Halpern uses his experience in *Wyatt v. Stickney* and other right-to-treatment litigation to focus on the recently renewed interest of the legal community in the rights of institutionalized citizens, especially the mentally retarded. Of particular concern to Halpern is the right of institutionalized patients to be dealt with as *citizens* and, more specifically, of the right of the mentally retarded to habilitation.

Question: Should resources available to the society for mental health be focused on the presently disabled, as called for in recent right-to-treatment cases, or focused on preventive efforts? Would we be better advised to focus on mental *health* or on the *cure* of mental *illness*? This important and long-argued value question provides one focus for Stuart Golann's chapter, "The Core Problem Controversy and the Right to Treatment."

Fremouw's summary chapter puts together many of the issues raised in discussion during the conference, including most importantly, the problem of evaluating standards on the basis of "input" variables such as were required by the court in *Wyatt v. Stickney* (i.e., number and training of staff, specification of physical facilities, and necessity for individualized treatment program) versus "output" variables (i.e., how well does the treatment work in returning patients to useful, productive, noninstitutionalized lives). Also of particular interest is the question: Does a voluntary patient have a right to treatment comparable to that of an involuntary patient? Ultimately, is mental health care as well as general health care a *right* of all citizens or only a *service* to be purchased by those with sufficient financial resources?

The conference and this resulting book provide an exciting beginning for the essential, professional and political discussion of issues involved in assuring an ultimate *right to mental health* by beginning here with the *right to treatment*.

A New Right to Treatment

WILLIAM J. FREMOUW

During the last decade, several court cases have challenged the adequacy of the care and treatment received in mental hospitals by patients involuntarily institutionalized. Within the last 3 years, the courts have heard cases arguing the right to adequate treatment for all, voluntary and involuntary, residents of mental institutions and institutions for the retarded.

The issue of the right to treatment is potentially the most significant in the mental health field today. Court decisions upholding the right of residents of institutions to receive adequate treatment may initiate major institutional changes. On the other hand, decisions may inadvertently perpetuate archaic institutional care in an era of slowly emerging advances from the past. This chapter by William Fremouw examines the historical and legal evolution of the right to treatment, the complexity of creating standards, and problems of enforcing this right.

THE RECOGNITION OF THE RIGHT TO TREATMENT

Early Right to Treatment Cases

In 1960, Morton Birnbaum proclaimed the advent of a new right to treatment for institutionalized citizens.[1] As summarized in an editorial:

The fact that a person has a mental ailment is not a crime. Therefore, if anyone is involuntarily restrained of his liberty because of a mental ailment, that state owes a duty to provide him reasonable medical attention. If medical attention reasonably well adapted to his needs is not given, the victim is not a patient but virtually a prisoner.[2]

7

Courts have traditionally overlooked the serious issues of civil liberty involved in involuntary commitment procedures. These hearings, which often result in lifelong institutional confinement, are euphemistically labeled "civil proceedings" for "rehabilitative hospitalization." Judicial hearings for involuntary commitment are sometimes as short as 1.6 minutes and average 8 minutes in several courts.[3] When confronted with an allegation of lack of treatment by a patient who is petitioning for release by writ of habeas corpus, the courts have supported continued confinement without making a real investigation, either on the ground that the petitioner is receiving treatment or on the ground that the court is not competent to judge the adequacy of treatment.

In California, for example, a state court rejected the plea of a "sexual psychopath" arrested for a minor offense that his lifetime incarceration "for treatment" in a penitentiary was a cruel punishment. The court stated that "the emphasis that appellant places on the fact that he was originally convicted of a misdemeanor and now finds himself in San Quentin, possibly for life, is misplaced. This argument would be sound only were his confinement *punishment*"[4] (emphasis added). No psychiatric treatment was demonstrated to exist for this man in prison. In another case, *Millard v. Cameron,*[5] a federal district court refused to hear the argument that an inmate of a mental hospital had only mopped floors and watched television for several years. The court stated that standards for evaluation of adequate treatment were beyond its judicial competence. Indefinitely committed as a sexual psychopath after being charged with exhibiting himself, a misdemeanor punishable by a 90 days' imprisonment, Millard faced indefinite confinement with little hope for treatment or release.

In other decisions courts hesitantly began to move toward the recognition of a right to treatment, first invoking semantic arguments. *In re Maddox,*[6] the court ruled that a person involuntarily committed as a sexual psychopath and not convicted of any crime may not be confined in a "penal" institution, although state psychiatrists testified that this treatment was prescribed to help the patient learn self-discipline. He was ordered returned to a mental hospital for treatment. In *Miller v. Overholser*[7] the court stated that a person who is not legally insane and involuntarily confined under a "remedial" sexual psychopath statute may not be kept in a place for "the hopeless and violent."[8] Confinement on a custodial ward with regressed, assaultive patients was declared a violation of the remedial spirit of the statute. Although the specific treatment was not explored in either case, the courts acted upon the right of these men to be confined in a situation that ostensibly provided psychiatric treatment.

In 1964, *Sas v. Maryland*[9] was the first case to examine a treatment program to determine whether the involuntary confinement met constitutional requirements. Sas, who had been committed under Maryland's Defective Delinquent Act,[10] asserted that his indeterminate sentence could not be justified because he was not receiving any treatment. The court remanded on constitutional issues including whether the institution furnished treatment for the "defective delinquents" sufficient to distinguish their incarceration from the confinement of other law breakers. Although the fourteenth amendment issue was raised, the case was resolved on the point that Sas was not a defective delinquent, without further consideration of his right to treatment.

The first case to directly address itself to the right to treatment and arouse national interest was *Rouse v. Cameron*[11] in 1966. The petitioner, Charles Rouse, had been committed to Saint Elizabeths Hospital, Washington, D.C., in 1962 after being found not guilty by reason of insanity of carrying a dangerous weapon, a misdemeanor with a 1-year maximum sentence. After 3 years of confinement, he petitioned for release by a writ of habeas corpus alleging that he had not received psychiatric treatment during his confinement. The court refused to hear the claim because of a lack of jurisdiction.[12] When the circuit court of appeals reviewed the case, Justice Bazelon's opinion echoed the editorial written 6 years earlier which first declared the right to treatment. "The purpose of involuntary hospitalization is treatment, not punishment. . . . Absent treatment, the hospital is transform[ed] . . . into a penitentiary where one could be held indefinitely for no convicted offense."[13]

The decision strongly implied that a constitutional right to treatment exists under the due process, equal protection, and cruel and unusual punishment clauses. The court stated:

Absence of treatment might draw into question the constitutionality of this mandatory commitment section. . . . It has also been suggested that failure to supply treatment may violate the equal protection clause. Indefinite confinement without treatment of one who has been found not criminally responsible may be so inhumane as to be "cruel and unusual punishment."[14]

However, the court merely raised the questions before reversing the lower court decision on statutory instead of constitutional grounds. The Hospitalization of the Mentally Ill Act,[15] which states a right to treatment for civilly committed mental patients, was interpreted to guarantee the right to adequate treatment to people found not guilty by reason of insanity. The court then remanded the case to the district court for a hearing to determine if Rouse was receiving adequate treatment.

This decision established the issue of adequate treatment as relevant in habeas corpus hearings. In addition, the court dictated that the right to treatment exists regardless of the institution's lack of facilities or staff. Citing civil rights cases as precedent, the court said "the rights here asserted are *present* rights . . . and, unless there is an overwhelming compelling reason, they are to be promptly fulfilled."[16] Although avoiding a decision on constitutional grounds, *Rouse* marked the real dawn of the right to treatment. The strong language of the decision forewarned the legal and medical profession of future decisions further establishing and expanding the right of institutionalized citizens to receive adequate treatment.

Rouse had been institutionalized after being found not guilty by reason of insanity. The next case raising the right to treatment was initiated by John Nason, an indicted murderer who had never been to trial.[17] After spending 5 years in Bridgewater State Hospital, Massachusetts, because of incompetency to stand trial, Nason petitioned for habeas corpus on the ground that the hospital was so understaffed that adequate psychiatric treatment was impossible. Nason claimed that treatment in Bridgewater was so inferior to other state institutions that his confinement denied him equal protection of the law. Taking an active interest in these allegations, the court appointed a special commissioner, whose opinion would be binding, to investigate the conditions at Bridgewater State Hospital. The commissioner's report confirmed Nason's charges of chronic understaffing at Bridgewater and inferior treatment relative to other hospitals. Since Nason was never convicted of a crime and his confinement was based on a nonpenal statute, the court said "it is necessary that the remedial aspects of confinement . . . have foundation in fact."[18] The court also concurred that Nason's "confinement might have deprived him of liberty without due process of law."[19] The court warned that if adequate treatment was not furnished within a reasonable time the legality of further confinement would be dubious. This decision began to imbed the right to treatment for involuntarily committed mental patients on the constitutional grounds of due process and equal protection of the law.

Class Action Suits for Adequate Treatment

As courts started to recognize constitutional grounds for adequate treatment, new cases began to reveal a strategically different use of the right to treatment that has a much greater impact on the mental health field. Instead of seeking release for an involuntarily committed individual from a nontreatment situation, cases beginning with *Wyatt v. Stickney*[20] argued for the implementation of adequate treatment for all residents of mental institutions and institutions for the retarded. The right-to-treatment argument is expanded from a point in a writ of habeas corpus suit to the basic assumption of class action suits by voluntary and involuntary residents and even staff of institutions to gain significant improvements in care.

In October 1970, a claim of inadequate treatment was made in a class action by the patients as well as staff of Alabama's Bryce Hospital in a suit *Wyatt v. Stickney*. Staff participation had been precipitated by the sudden firing of 99 hospital employees because of a budget reduction. The suit sought an injunction against the state to rescind the dismissal of the employees, to forbid further admissions to the hospital, and to guarantee the continued care of the hospital patients. The suit alleged that the consitutional rights of the involuntarily committed patients were violated by the inadequate treatment they received. At the time of the suit, the hospital was being reorganized into a unit system which had not been fully implemented. The court declined to evaluate the treatment provided by the new unitization program. However, it did evaluate the treatment received by the involuntarily committed patients prior to the reorganization. Declared completely inadequate, the treatment did not meet any minimum standard for treatment of the mentally ill. With that finding, the U. S. district court was the first federal court to unequivocally establish the constitutional right of the involuntarily committed to receive adequate treatment. (*Rouse* had intimated the constitutional right but based the decision on a statutory right to treatment. In *Nason*, a state court had stated the constitutional right.) Judge Johnson said:

[there was no possible] legal [or moral] justification for the state of Alabama's failing to afford treatment . . . to the several thousand patients who have been civilly committed . . . for treatment purposes. To deprive any citizen of his or her liberty upon the altruistic theory that the confinement is for humane therapeutic reasons and then fail to provide adequate treatment violates the very fundamentals of due process.[21]

This is a very important decision because it established precedent for future federal court decisions. In addition, the right to treatment for the involuntarily committed exists despite an Alabama statute exercising police power to commit individuals just "for safekeeping."[22] Due process must be satisfied if people are involuntarily committed for treatment by state *parens patriae* power and do not receive treatment. Although no promise of treatment is implied in the term "safekeeping," this decision established that a promise of treatment is implicit in any involuntary commitment statute. When a state deprives a mentally ill person of his liberty that state must provide due process. In this context, due process is beginning to be in the form of a right to effective treatment.

In August 1971, the right to treatment for the mentally retarded was first presented in court. The court granted a motion to amend *Wyatt* to include residents of Searcy Hospital and Partlow State School for the Retarded in the class of plaintiffs currently denied their constitutional rights to treatment. Recognizing the major questions of civil rights involved in the case, the court asked for the assistance of the U. S. Justice Department to investigate the conditions at Partlow State School. After receiving the findings of a 3-week investigation by a team of six FBI agents, Judge Johnson described Partlow State School as "a warehousing institution which, because of its atmosphere of psychological and physical deprivation, is wholly incapable of furnishing treatment of the mentally retarded and is conducive only to the deterioration and the debilitation of the residents."[23]

Upon these findings the court concluded that the residents had been denied their right to habilitation. ("Habilitation" is the process by which trained personnel, including psychologists, physicians, and educators, assist the mentally retarded to acquire and maintain life skills.[24]) The court stated that because "the only constitutional justification for civilly committing a mental retardate, therefore, is habilitation, it follows ineluctably that once committed such a person is possessed of an inviolable constitutional right to habilitation."[25]

This decision first recognized the right to treatment for the involuntarily committed mentally retarded. However, the court failed to consider the significant issue of the right to treatment for the voluntarily committed mentally retarded. Assuming that all residents were involuntarily committed because no evidence was presented in rebuttal, the court left this issue for future courts to decide.[26]

As precedent-setting as the affirmation of a constitutional right to treatment for involuntarily committed mental patients and mental retardates was the judicial action to enforce a right to treatment. Judge Johnson's initial response to the evidence of inadequate treatment at Bryce Hospital was similar to action in *Nason*—wait and see. Since the hospital was in the process of reorganization, Bryce officials were given 6 months to make necessary improvements to provide proper treatment.[27] In *Nason*, the hospital easily could provide treatment for one person within a reasonable time. However, in a class action suit, not just one but everyone in the institution requires adequate treatment to satisfy court orders. Six months later the court ruled that the state had failed to implement a treatment program satisfying minimum medical and constitutional standards. Treatment was declared inadequate in three fundamental areas: the hospital failed to provide (1) a humane psychological and physical environment; (2) qualified staff in sufficient numbers to administer adequate treatment; and (3) individualized treatment plans.[28]

A few months later, after hearing testimony of the urgency of the need for treatment at Partlow State School, the court made the first major judicial intervention into the mental health field. By the Interim Emergency Order, the hiring of 300 additional workers within 30 days, immunization of all residents within 10 days, and complete review and revision of all drug prescriptions within 15 days was ordered by Justice Johnson.[29]

The most significant court ruling in the evolution of the right to treatment occurred April 13, 1972. The court had invited several national organizations to assist the court as amici curiae. Amici, the American Association of Mental Deficiency, the American Psychological Association, the American Orthopsychiatric Association and the American Civil Liberties Union, recommended standards for the operation of the three institutions necessary to provide adequate treatment. After the 3-day hearing, extensive changes in the Alabama institutions were ordered. This final ruling specified standards for every aspect of institutional care, from a minimum of 206.5 staff members for 250 mentally ill patients, to acceptable temperatures for hot water, to individualized treatment plans for each resident.[30] Anticipating fiscal arguments against fulfilling the new standards for care, the court ruled that "the unavailability of neither funds, nor staff nor facilities, will justify a default by defendants in the provision of suitable treatment."[31] The court has reserved ruling on the plaintiffs' motion to appoint a master to oversee the implementation of the orders and to direct the sale of portions of the extensive land holdings of the Mental Health Board, or to place an injunction against the treasurer and comptroller of the state to authorize nonessential state spending. The court deferred the administration and fiscal implementation of this order to the responsible government bodies but may later order these steps if necessary to assure adequate care.[32] The Minimum Standards for Adequate Care and Treatment are included in the Source Material.

The State of Alabama has appealed this decision to the United States court of appeals to challenge the federal district court's jurisdiction over the case. Alabama argues that an involuntary commitment does not require treatment. "The primary purpose and justification for commitment of persons who are mentally ill is not their 'cure' but is avoidance of the injury which they might inflict upon themselves or others if they are not confined."[33] From this reasoning, Alabama concludes that no constitutional issues are raised to give a federal court jurisdiction. The appeal decision will decide the constitutionality of a right to treatment of the individual as derived from states' role as *parens patriae* or the states' police power to protect society. If protection of society is a sufficient basis for involuntary commitment, civil commitment procedures will probably satisfy the due process constitutional requirement. However, if the court decides that involuntary commitment is predicated upon treatment of the individual, then adequate treatment may be necessary to satisfy due process and create federal jurisdiction over a constitutional issue.

The class action format, the broad decisions on constitutional grounds, the extensive use of ancillary expert advice, and the forceful use of judicial power in *Wyatt* may mark the advent of an enforced right to treatment. Other suits have already followed.

In Massachusetts, *Ricci v. Greenblatt*[34] is a class action suit initiated by a group of parents for their mentally retarded children institutionalized at Belchertown State School. The complaint stated that "the conditions in which the plaintiffs and the class they represent live are so shockingly oppressive, unsanitary, unhealthy and degrading that they are an affront to basic human decency and a violation of fundamental constitutional rights."[35] The complaint cites ample evidence to support the charges. A special legislative report in 1970 intimated that residents at Belchertown are denied equal protection of the law by the inequitable distribution of resources among state institutions. In fiscal year 1969, $3,100 was expended for each resident at Belchertown while $3,600 was spent for each resident at a similar state institution, Fernald State School. Another report in March 1971 by the Joint Special Commission of Belchertown State School and Manson State School was quoted as further evidence of the inadequate treatment prevalent at Belchertown. Among the statements, the Commission Report said:

In some buildings at Belchertown excrement and urine are constantly visible and unattended . . . cockroaches have . . . overrun several buildings to the extent of crawling over immobile patients . . . parts of the living quarters at Belchertown are in violation of the State Sanitary Code . . . there is no semblance of privacy at Belchertown . . . punishment has bordered on cruel and abusive treatment . . . prescribed medical care is delayed or ignored for long periods of time. . . . The education, vocational education and recreation staff are insufficient and cannot provide realistic services for the school population.[36]

The suit argues that (1) the oppressive physical environment marked by overcrowded, deteriorating structures, (2) the lack of dental, medical or educational treatment programs, and (3) the regimented, impersonal environment of brutality and dehumanization created by staff shortages clearly violate many constitutional rights. The failure to provide adequate medical and other professional treatment discriminates against the mentally retarded institutionalized residents and violates the guarantee of equal protection of the law. The denial of access to telephone, mail and attorneys, their basic civil liberties, represents punishment without trial in violation of due process of law. The conditions at Belchertown are alleged to deny the right to be treated with decency and dignity and accorded privacy guaranteed by the fourteenth amendment. In addition, the living conditions and the lack of treatment and care constitute cruel and abusive punishment.[37]

On February 11, 1972, a federal court issued a restraining order to prohibit transfer or admission until "adequate treatment and humane living conditions exist." Complete medical evaluation and comprehensive treatment plans for all residents were ordered and a freeze on staff hiring was revoked.[38] The court retained jurisdiction of the case to assure fulfillment of the orders.

Two weeks later the State of Massachusetts motioned to dismiss the case from federal court because of lack of jurisdiction. The state contended that "a constitutional right to treatment cannot be predicated upon a system of voluntary admission."[39] Because mental health laws had been recently revised to eliminate the involuntary commitment of mental retardates, all the residents are voluntarily institutionalized.[40] In all previous cases, i.e., *Rouse, Nason, Wyatt,* a constitutional right to treatment was recognized in the context of involuntary noncriminal confinement. The State of Massachusetts contended that because residency at Belchertown was "voluntary," the complaint concerns only the adequacy of a state-provided service, not a constitutional issue under federal jurisdiction. The court rejected this motion without giving an opinion.[41] The restraining order and the denial of the state's motion tacitly signify the federal court's recognition of a right to treatment for voluntary residents of institutions for the retarded. The defendants filed an answer to the original complaint on April 20, 1972, denying each allegation outlined in the 46-page complaint.

Over 18 months later, on November 12, 1973, a consent decree for specific improvements at Belchertown State School was signed between the state and plaintiffs. After 6 months of intensive negotiation lead by U. S. District Court Judge Tauro, the state agreed to seek a $2.6 million state bond for improvements to 22 buildings as well as hire 80 additional domestic workers and 36 new professional staff.[42] This legal agreement represents a significant contrast with the adversarial atmosphere of *Wyatt* where the state opposed the suit and appealed the decision. Although the *Ricci* suit has not yet produced a definitive court decision on the right of voluntary patients to receive treatment, the negotiated consent decree establishes a new precedent for disposition of cases in which involved parties under court direction attempt to evolve a feasible plan for progress.

Within a few months after *Ricci* was initiated, in New York and Georgia other suits had begun to further test the constitutionality of a right to treatment. In March 1972, a class action suit for the 5,200 residents of Willowbrook State School was filed in New York federal district court by the New York Association for Retarded Children, alleging that the institution does not meet minimum constitutional standards of adequate habilitation. Overcrowding, inadequate staffing, inhumane living conditions, no school for 80 percent of the school-age residents and improper medical treatment at the institution were cited as denying the mentally retarded their constitutional rights under the first, fourth, fifth, sixth, eighth, thirteenth and fourteenth amendments. Echoing some constitutional arguments from *Wyatt* to *Ricci,* this suit expanded the constitutional issues to include allegations of involuntary servitude by residents involuntarily required to work in the institution which violates the thirteenth amendment's abolition of slavery.

The court was requested to: (1) hold a hearing to determine minimum standards for the operation of Willowbrook; (2) then issue an injunction to direct state compliance with these standards; and (3) appoint a master to oversee the implementation of the court ruling. The plaintiffs and defendants were scheduled to meet to begin to develop minimum standards.[43]

In response New York State initiated a massive hiring program to replace the 600 employees that Willowbrook State School had lost by attrition since December, 1970 when a statewide hiring freeze was initiated. Plans were drawn for up to 1,500 jobs to be filled to help relieve manpower shortages at Willowbrook and five other understaffed state institutions. Motivated by public concern stimulated by extensive television coverage of the conditions at Willowbrook, the state announced that $5 million in fiscal year 1972, $12.4 million in fiscal year 1973, and $25 million in 1974 will be available to improve inadequate staffing and overcrowding at its institutions for the retarded. A three-phase program to accomplish both short-term and long-range goals for the care and treatment of the retarded was developed.[44]

On April 10, 1973, the federal district court returned a decision that ordered New York State to take nine specific steps to correct shortages of personnel, establish a contract with an accredited hospital, repair toilets, and to submit periodic progress reports to the court. A significant aspect of the decision was Judge Judd's rejection of the plaintiffs' contention that a constitutional right to treatment or rehabilitation exists. Instead, federal jurisdiction was based on the courts' responsibility to protect the retarded from harm.[45] This decision, while continuing to assert judicial power over the care of institutionalized people, modified the grounds of authority from protecting an affirmative right to adequate treatment established in *Wyatt* to protecting people from harm without affirming the existence of more than nondebilitating conditions.

In Georgia, the state fought a right-to-treatment suit filed March 29, 1972, on behalf of all residents in Georgia's six mental health and mental retardation facilities. The class action suit alleged that the State of Georgia is violating the fifth, eighth, and fourteenth amendments to the Constitution in the care of the institutional resident. The complaint sought a precedent-setting court ruling that all institutional residents, voluntary or involuntary, mentally ill or retarded, have a right to adequate treatment. The establishment of minimum constitutional standards for treatment and the development of effective individualized treatment plans were sought by the plaintiffs. A federal district court dismissed the case on the ground that a constitutional right to treatment does not exist.[46] The *Burnham v. Department of Public Health of the State of Georgia* decision was appealed by the plaintiffs and consolidated with the *Wyatt v. Stickney* appeal. This direct contradiction between district courts will be arbitrated by the Fifth Circuit Court of Appeals' decision on the cases.

Although the Fifth Circuit had not yet decided the issues presented in *Wyatt* and *Burnham*, a federal district court in Minnesota has made a new decision on the threshold legal issues raised by the right-to-treatment cases. In the case of *Welsch v. Likins*,[47] involuntarily committed residents of schools for the retarded in Minnesota brought a class action against the state to receive adequate treatment. In the most scholarly ruling among right-to-treatment cases, Judge Larson thoroughly examined and discussed the underlying constitutional issues in right to treatment, including the contradictions between the *Wyatt* and *Burnham* cases. A lengthy decision issued February 15, 1974 rejected the arguments in the *Burnham* decision, expanded the ruling in the *Willowbrook* case, and reaffirmed that a constitutional right to treatment exists under the due process clause of the fourteenth amendment first established in *Wyatt*. Consistant with *Wyatt*, Larson ruled that care and treatment are required *quid pro quo* liberty for involuntary commitment. After thus establishing federal jurisdiction, the merits of the particular case will be heard. This decision appears in the Source Materials.

Related Class Action Suits

Institutionalized residents are not the only group contesting their treatment. The format of the right-to-treatment suits, class actions seeking adequate treatment on legal and constitutional grounds, has been generalized to right-to-education suits on behalf of retarded and emotionally disturbed children residing in the community. In Louisiana, *Lebanks v. Spears*[48] is a class action by children labelled mentally retarded and denied any form of special education without a hearing or right to appeal. The complaint seeks an injunction to guarantee the opportunity to receive special education geared to special needs for all children residing in the community. The *Coalition for the Civil Rights of Handicapped Persons v. the State of Michigan*[49] is a class action alleging that children excluded from public schools because of mental, behavioral, physical or emotional handicaps are denied publicly supported education and receive only custodial care, a violation of the equal protection and due process clause of the fourteenth amendment. The class action *Mills v. Board of Education of the District of Columbia* on August 1, 1972 established the right of all children to receive education. The plaintiffs, who had been denied public schooling because of alleged mental, behavioral, physical or emotional handicaps or deficiencies, won this right on the constitutional grounds that denial of public education to "exceptional" children without a hearing, right to appeal or alternative educational opportunities violates the due process clause of the fifth amendment.[50]

In addition to the right to education, class actions are beginning to test the right to rehabilitation in prisons. In *Holt v. Sarver,* a class action against the Arkansas prison system, the court began to question if a constitutional basis for rehabilitation may exist. In cautious language reminiscent of early right-to-treatment decisions, the court states: "The absence of an affirmative program of training and rehabilitation may have a constitutional significance where in the absence of such a program conditions and practices exist which militate against reform and rehabilitation."[51]

Other courts have also implied a constitutional basis for state delivery of constructive programs for prisoners instead of mere incarceration. The Supreme Court of Pennsylvania found that the lack of rehabilitative programs producing forced inactivity combined with other substandard prison conditions could constitute cruel and unusual punishment.[52] At present, prisons are not required to provide educational and vocational programs to inmates. However, these class actions have established that states are responsible to prevent conditions that make rehabilitation difficult to achieve. Other class action suits have already been initiated to more positively affirm a right to rehabilitation in prisons.

These suits and others are beginning to test the right of all citizens, regardless of their handicap or residency, to receive care, treatment and education at the level required to be humane and constructive. The continued second-class citizenship of our silent, forgotten, impaired children and adults, perpetuated by public apathy and insufficient funds, is being challenged.

To summarize, the right to treatment remained a dormant force cautiously hinted at by a few judicial decisions during the first 6 years of the 1960's. *Rouse* in 1966 and then *Nason* marked the real birth of a recognized right to receive adequate institutional care. With *Wyatt* a metamorphosis began that has transformed the right to treatment into a potential weapon for major institutional and societal change in the treatment of handicapped citizens. The power of this new weapon is being tested across the country. We have only just begun to see the effects of the legal intervention into the mental health system and other human services precipitated by the right to treatment.

STANDARDS FOR ADEQUATE TREATMENT

The recognition of a right to treatment necessitates the establishment of standards to evaluate treatment received. The development of standards evolved as the right to treatment matured in the courts. In early cases the court was loathe to consider the adequacy of the treatment of an individual. Instead, the court in *Daniels,*[53] for example, considered only whether the institution as a whole was totally ineffectual in treatment, completely ignoring allegations of inadequate treatment for the individual.

Rouse v. Cameron[54] first established judicial standards to evaluate adequacy of treatment. Judge Bazelon stated that the hospital need not show that treatment will cure or improve him but only that there is a bonafide effort to do so, and thus requires the hospital to show that initial and periodic inquiries are made into needs and conditions of the patient with view to providing suitable treatment for him, and that the program provided is suited to his particular needs.[55]

Adequate treatment is defined as a program designed to the needs of a particular patient and periodically reviewed and revised. The treatment must be adequate in the light of present knowledge. The possibility of a better treatment does not necessarily prove that the present program is inadequate.[56]

This opinion aroused a storm of criticism and skepticism over the competence of courts to protect a right to treatment. Members of the medical profession warned that given radically different psychiatric opinions about types of treatment, judges will have little basis to choose among varieties of treatment. The American Psychiatric Association issued an official policy statement in response to *Rouse*. They said that "the definition of treatment and the appraisal of its adequacy are matters for medical determination."[57] In addition to asserting a professional monopoly on the evaluation of adequate treatment, they maintain treatment must be evaluated relative to *available* staff and resources, and not relative to any set of minimum standards for staffing or resources.[58] This very defensive policy would maintain the current levels of inadequate treatment across the country.

Legal commentators have also expressed their concerns over the enforcement of the right to treatment. The *Harvard Law Review* bemoaned "the difficulty of formulating standards of adequacy seems very great."[59] Morton Birnbaum, the physician-lawyer who first proclaimed a right to treatment, cautiously argued for the use of objective standards such as institutional accreditation and a minimum number of physician consultations and examinations as criteria for evaluation of the adequacy of treatment.[60] These criteria are proposed for the pragmatic value of saving professional time in court appearances to testify about the treatment of a particular individual. Although the use of limited professional manpower is a valid issue, the proposal that institutional standards alone should determine adequacy of treatment naively ignores individual needs of patients. Minimum staff ratios and doctor consultations are necessary but are not sufficient to guarantee that correct treatment is being provided. Within institutions, great variability in staff and resources often exist on different wards. The use of just institutional standards to evaluate adequacy of treatment could easily produce token observance of the right to treatment by an accredited institution that may not be providing individualized, quality care for particular patients.

Judge Bazelon has defended the courts' ability to enforce standards for adequate treatment. Courts have often supervised technical areas such as railroad rates, airplane designs or dam building without expert knowledge in the particular area. Not purporting to be a psychiatric expert, Bazelon defines an administrative role for the court. "The judge must decide only whether the patient is receiving carefully chosen therapy which respectable professional opinion regards as within the range of appropriate treatment alternatives, not whether the patient is receiving the best of all possible treatment in the best of all possible mental hospitals."[61]

The concept of adequate treatment must function at both the institutional and individual levels. In *Rouse,* treatment standards were established at the level of the individual. In addition, an institution must possess the physical facilities, staff and resources to meet minimum standards for adequate care. Obviously, a hospital cannot provide adequate treatments for any given patient if it lacks the resources to furnish any treatment. Also the ability of a hospital to provide treatment does not insure the delivery of proper individual treatment. Individual treatment must be evaluated in reference to individual needs. Minimum institutional standards, the presence of an individualized treatment plan consistent with current professional knowledge, and continued supervision and reevaluation of the treatment by qualified professionals are necessary for adequate treatment as set forth in *Rouse*.

Class action suits present a larger problem of evaluation of adequate treatment for the court. The evaluation of the treatment received by thousands, not just one, becomes the court's duty. In *Wyatt,*[62] hearings were conducted at which nationally recognized experts in mental retardation and mental illness proposed standards for adequate treatment. The court ordered standards and established criteria at the institutional level such as minimum staff ratios, and criteria at the individual level such as individualized treatment plans and reviews as necessary for adequate treatment.

At first consideration, the 206.5 personnel for every 250 patients required by *Wyatt* appears to furnish sufficient personnel for adequate treatment. However, what type of treatment can the type of staff required provide? These judicial standards are distinctively lower than the ratio of one psychiatrist, one psychologist and one social worker recommended by amici for every 30–50 patients.[63] The type of treatment mandated by the *Wyatt* staffing standards appears to only fortify a medical-custodial model of treatment where primarily psychiatric aides and nurses provide the direct care under the assumptions and supervision of medical professionals. The goal of establishing standards for adequate therapeutic treatment may have alluded the comprehensive *Wyatt* standards.

In spite of the medical model of treatment dictated by *Wyatt* standards, a recent article of the *American Journal of Psychiatry* urgently restated a fear of judicial intervention into traditionally medical affairs. Jonas Robitscher told his fellow physicians: "We can recognize that there is a right to treatment. We can also insist that courts use simple yardsticks—which *psychiatry* will have to develop quickly—to help the legal determination of treatment adequacy from usurping *psychiatric* authority and determining hospital policy" (emphasis added).[64]

After decades of medical treatment and authority dominating institutional care, others hold that perhaps new models of treatment and all mental health professions may combine to justly displace psychiatric authority and attempt to finally deliver adequate treatment to our institutionalized citizens. Future judicial decisions will undoubtedly maintain the need for individualized treatment. Equally certain, the *Wyatt* institutional standards will serve as a basis for future debates over questions of resources, manpower and models of treatment.

ENFORCEMENT OF THE RIGHT TO TREATMENT

Establishing standards for adequate treatment requires the ability to enforce the standards. The judiciary possesses several options to effect adequate care. In cases of involuntarily committed patients, a writ of habeas corpus requires the court to determine if the original commitment procedures were satisfied and if adequate treatment implicit in the commitment statutes has been furnished. Judges are empowered with four alternative actions: (1) deny the petition; (2) order immediate release of the petitioner; (3) order release of the petitioner if treatment is not improved; or (4) transfer the petitioner to a more appropriate institution. Birnbaum advocates that courts immediately release the petitioner if treatment has not been provided. Although the release of a mentally ill person who may require further treatment may endanger society and the person, he argues that the release of a patient denied adequate treatment would educate society to its constitutional obligation to provide treatment for its citizens involuntarily committed to institutions. Society could remove this potential danger by providing the adequate treatment necessary.[65] However, a writ of habeas corpus would not benefit the growing group of individuals who seek treatment and not release.

Other options less dramatic than immediate release from institutions are available. In situations where the petitioner has not been given treatment equal to what others receive in the same institution, a court mandamus could compel a superintendent to cease any discrimination against the person and furnish proper care. However, because the court cannot provide funds necessary to furnish adequate care, a mandamus is limited to the few situations in which care is available but undelivered.[66]

One of the most potent judicial remedies to enforce a right to treatment is the power to award monetary damages from the state for confinement in a nontreatment institution. In *Whitree v. State*,[67] the plaintiff was committed to a state hospital after being found incompetent to stand trial. Whitree spent 14 years in a New York State hospital without receiving adequate psychiatric care. The court found that his hospital record lacked both medical examinations and a treatment plan. It stated that "if that man had received proper and adequate psychiatric treatment such diagnosis [of sanity] would have been developed much sooner: and Whitree would have been released from Matteawan State Hospital much sooner."[68] Supporting Whitree's claim of false imprisonment for the majority of his confinement, the court awarded him $300,000 in damages from the state. The widespread judicial recognition of the right to damages in tort for inadequate care could be staggering. It cost New York State more money to repay Whitree than to have provided him with the best psychiatric treatment available in the world. Awards of $300,000 may stimulate legislative reform of institutions as an economic measure to avoid more costly suits. The right to damages in tort is based on charges of false imprisonment of the involuntarily committed and cannot apply to the voluntarily committed. When faced with class action suits, direct judicial action into institutional care by temporary restraining orders and injunctions has been used. The power of the court has even ordered such major changes in institutional care as the hiring of 300 employees in Alabama.

Although this overview of the judicial arsenal to enforce a right to treatment is impressive, the real potential to implement and maintain adequate treatment resides with the state legislatures' power to appropriate funds and to write comprehensive mental health legislation. One potential legislative role to support the right to treatment is the establishment of a policy-making and enforcement agency to guarantee adequate treatment. In Pennsylvania, "The Right to Treatment Law of 1968"[69] was the first attempt by any legislature to regulate the important problems of adequate care for inmates of public mental institutions. The bill proposed the establishment of a Mental Treatment Standards Committee to draft institutional criteria for adequate treatment such as minimum personnel-patient ratios. A different body, a Patient Treatment Review Board, would investigate, hear and decide questions of adequate treatment. If inadequate treatment is found, a 3-month period to improve treatment is given the institution. After that time, the patient may seek release through a court hearing. The bill prohibits the adoption of any specific requirements for methods or quality of treatment and states that no patient has a right to any particular quality of treatment. The Pennsylvania General Assembly failed to enact the statute during its 1968 session.[70]

This initial effort to legislate administrative machinery to guarantee adequate treatment contained several practical limitations. In this bill, a patient must take the initiative to raise a question of adequate treatment. Instead, a periodic review of all patients would more fairly insure adequate treatment for all patients, not just those well informed and motivated to challenge the adequacy of their treatment. In addition, the proposed review board did not possess any power to order and enforce an effective remedy such as discharge of the patient. The courts would still be burdened with such procedures. The major weakness of the bill is the absence of any standards for the Patient Review Board to evaluate the quality of individual care. As proposed earlier, the existence of a periodically reviewed and revised individual treatment plan supervised by a mental health professional should be a minimum requirement for adequate care. Future legislation rectifying these weaknesses would begin to insure adequate treatment.

The legislation of standards and administrative agencies to guarantee adequate treatment is one effort to resolve the problem of inadequate treatment of this nation's institutionalized mental patients and retardates. However, the most critical legislative role to insure adequate treatment is the appropriation of sufficient resources to provide proper care. The conditions reported in Alabama and Massachusetts reveal that the creation of a review board cannot remove the years of neglect and deterioration present in many institutions. Legislative concern and action is necessary to create real treatment. However, even legislative and public concern and money are not panaceas for all the ailments and blights accompanying institutionalization of mental patients and retardates.

NOTES

1. M. Birnbaum, "The Right to Treatment," *American Bar Association Journal,* 46 (1960), 499-503.

2. Editorial, "A New Right," *American Bar Association Journal,* 46 (1960), 516-17

3. T. Scheff, "Social Conditions for Rationality: How Urban and Rural Courts Deal with the Mentally Ill," *American Behavioral Scientist,* 7 (March 1964), 21-27.

4. People v. Levy, 151 Cal. App. 2d 460, 311, P. 2d. 897 (1st Dist. Ct. App. 1957) at 902.

5. Millard v. Cameron, 373 F.2d 468 (D. C. Cir. 1966)

6. In Re Maddox, 351 Mich. 358, 88 N.W. 2d 470 (1958).

7. Miller v. Overholser, 206 F.2d 415 (D. C. Cir. 1953).

8. *Id.* at 419.

9. Sas v. Maryland, 334 F.2d 506 (4th Cir. 1964).

10. *Md. Ann. Code* art. 31B, 5 (1957).

11. Rouse v. Cameron, 373 F.2d 451 (D. C. Cir. 1966).

12. *Id.* at 452.

13. *Id.* at 453.

14. *Id.* at 453.

15. *D. C. Code Ann.* 21-801 (Supp. V. 1966).

16. Rouse v. Cameron, 373 F.2d 358 (D. C. Cir. 1966).

17. Nason v. Superintendent of Bridgewater State Hospital, 223 N. E. 2d 908 (Ma. 1968).

18. *Id.* at 913.

19. *Id.* at 908.

20. Wyatt v. Stickney, 325 F. Supp. 781 (M. D. Ala. 1971).

21. *Id.* at 785.

22. *Ala. Code* tit 45, 210 (1958).

23. Wyatt v. Stickney, C. A. 3195-N (M. D. Ala.), Unreported Interim Emergency Order of March 2, 1972.

24. Wyatt v. Stickney. C. A. 3195-N, (M. D. Ala.), Post Trial Memorandum of Amici at 5.

25. Wyatt v. Stickney, C. A. 3195-N (M. D. Ala), Order and Decree of April 13, 1972 at 4.

26. Id at 3.

27. Wyatt v. Stickney, 325 F. Supp. at 785.

28. Wyatt v. Stickney, C. A. 3195-N (M. D. Ala, Dec. 10, 1972), Court Report cited April 13, 1972 at 2.

29. Wyatt v. Stickney, C. A. 3195-N (M. D. Ala.), Unreported Interim Emergency Order of March 2, 1972.

30. Wyatt v. Stickney, C. A. 3195-N (M. D. Ala.), Appendix A. Order and Decree of April 13, 1972.

31. *Id.* at 5.

32. *Id.* at 6.

33. Wyatt v. Stickney, C. A. 3195-N (M. D. Ala.), Brief for Appellant, Oct. 18, 1972 at 11.

34. Ricci v. Greenblatt, C. A. No. 72-469-F (D. Mass., filed Feb. 7, 1972).

35. *Id.* at 7.

36. *Id.* at 11-13.

37. Id. at 43.

38. Ricci v. Greenblatt, C. A. No. 72-469-F (D. Mass.), Order of Feb. 11, 1972.

39. Ricci v. Greenblatt, C. A. No. 72-469-F (D. Mass.), Memorandum of March 1, 1972.

40. *Mass. Gen. Law* Ch. 123,S888(1971).

41. Ricci v. Greenblatt, C. A. No. 72-469-F (D. Mass.), Order of March 13, 1972.

42. P. Brunelle, "Battle of Belchertown Is Won by Parents," Springfield Union, November 13, 1973, pp. 1-2.

43. "Willowbrook Faces Class Action," *New Directions,* 2, No. 5 (May 1972), 2.

44. "N. Y. responds to Willowbrook Controversy," *New Directions,* 2, No. 5 (May 1972), 2.

45. New York State Association for Retarded Children, Inc. v. Rockefeller, 357 F. Supp. 752, 758 (E. D. N. Y. 1973).

46. Burnham v. Georgia, 349 F. Supp. 1335 (N. D. Ga. 1972).

47. Welsch v. Likins, C. A. No. 4-72-Civ. 451 (D. Minn.), Order and Decree Feb. 15, 1974.

48. Lebanks v. Spears, C. A. No. 71-2897 (E. D. La.), filed May 10, 1972.

49. Coalition v. State of Michigan, C. A. No. 38357 (E. D. Mich.), filed May 25, 1972.

50. Mills v. Board of Education of the District of Columbia, C. A. No. 1969-71 (D. D. C.), filed August 1, 1972.

51. Holt v. Sarver, 209 F. Supp. 362 (E. D. Ark. 1970), *aff'd,* 442 F. 2d 204 (8th Cir. 1971).

52. Commonwealth ex real. Bryant v. Hendrick, 44 Pa. 83 (1971).

53. Director of Patuxent Institute v. Daniels, 343 Md. 16, 221, A. 2d 426 (1966).

54. Rouse v. Cameron, 373 F. 2d 451 (D. C. Cir. 1966).

55. *Id.* at 457.

56. *Id..*

57. "Council of the American Psychiatric Association Position Statement on the Question of Adequacy of Treatment," *American Journal of Psychiatry,* 123 (1967), 1458-60.

58. *Id.* at 1460.

59. *Harvard Law Review,* 80 (1967), 898-900.

60. M. Birnbaum, "A Rationale for the Right," in *The Right to Treatment,* D. Burris (ed.) (New York: Springer Pub., 1969), pp. 79-80.

61. D. Bazelon, "Implementing the Right to Treatment," *University of Chicago Law Review*, 36 (1969), 742-801.

62. Wyatt v. Stickney, C. A. No. 3195-N (M. D. Ala.), Order and Decree of April 13, 1972.

63. Wyatt v. Stickney, C. A. No. 3195-N (M. D. Ala.), Pre-Trial Memorandum.

64. J. Robitscher, "Courts, State Hospitals, and the Right to Treatment," *American Journal of Psychiatry*, 129 (Sept. 1972), 79.

65. M. Birnbaum, "Implementing the Right to Treatment," *University of Chicago Law Review*, 36 (1969), 745.

66. "Nascent Right to Treatment," *Virginia Law Review*, 53 (1967), 1157-61.

67. Whitree v. State, Misc. 2d 693, 290 N. Y. S. 2d 486 (Ct. Cl. 1968).

68. *Id.* at 706, 290 N. Y. S. 2d, at 500.

69. S. B. 1274 and H.B. 2118, Pa. Gen. Ass., 1968 Session

70. Birnbaum, *supra* note 60, at 89.

EDITORS' NOTE: This chapter, in slightly altered form, appeared in *The Journal of Psychiatry and Law*, 2, No. 1 (Spring 1974), 7-31.

Wyatt v. Stickney: Background and Postscript

STONEWALL B. STICKNEY

The unique perspective of a psychiatrist interested in improving mental health services and himself serving as Commissioner of Mental Health at the time of the *Wyatt v. Stickney* lawsuit is provided by Stonewall Stickney in the following chapter. After providing a historical background for the state's mental health system, Dr. Stickney shares the problems, dilemmas and frustrations he faced when the case *Wyatt v. Stickney* made Alabama the first legal and political battleground of the expanded right to treatment. This commentary ends by raising several searching questions about strategies for change in the mental health system, the problems of creating standards of treatment and the potential paradoxical effect of the right to treatment in progress in mental health toward community alternatives to institutions.

BACKGROUND

In this country prior to the crusade of Dorothea Dix in the 1840's mentally ill and mentally retarded people were rarely regarded as the responsibility of the state in the sense of their being entitled by their condition to humane, compassionate and therapeutic treatment at public expense. The success of the Dorothea Dix crusade was memorialized in the construction of the state-supported public mental hospitals all over the nation. In the flush of 19th-century idealism it was anticipated that these asylums would provide modern, informed, humane treatment for the insane. For a couple of generations, considering the knowledge and the expectation of that day, they succeeded. For example, Alabama, a small frontier state in the 1860's, produced Bryce Hospital. In those days Bryce was an example to the nation because of its abolition of shackles and restraints, and its generally humane treatment of patients. Its first superintendent, Dr. Peter Bryce, also believed in the therapeutic efficacy of work. He could not anticipate that with public and legislative neglect patient labor would become the necessary economic base of the institution, i.e., that work therapy would become peonage. As early as 1875, however, Dr. Bryce was complaining that the original purpose of the hospital was being subverted by the involuntary commitment of paupers, old people, the mentally defective and harmless eccentrics or vagrants. He and his successors had difficulty stemming the tide of inappropriate referrals: they were contesting a developing "gentleman's agreement" by which physicians, judges and families found it convenient to ship unwanted people off to the state hospital. The county almshouses, poorfarms and old folks' homes were concomitantly disappearing, with a shift away from local county responsibility.

The late 19th-century prestige of Bryce Hospital, and others like it, could not long withstand overcrowding, fiscal starvation and progressive deterioration of buildings. Low pay, poor working conditions and a generally stagnant and pessimistic atmosphere in the state hospitals made it increasingly difficult to attract competent physicians, much less trained psychiatrists, psychologists and social workers.

The failure of most states and of the federal government (until the 1960's) to take the responsibility for decent treatment of the mentally ill was matched by the unconcern of the medical schools, centers of psychiatric training and organized psychiatry. In the medical schools, until recently, psychiatry was treated with condescension or derision by many of the faculty.

In the psychiatric residences the major effort was, and still is, to turn out private practitioners and a few academic and research psychiatrists. Extremely few psychiatrists have chosen to work in state mental departments or in state mental hospitals. Those who have done so have developed socioeconomic and political concerns so foreign to the everyday issues of private practice and academic psychiatry as to require a separate journal, organization and meetings.

While state and national public health systems were progressing well and public health was being taught in medical schools as a specialty, the major public health problem of this century, mental illness, was being ignored.

Most states were and are still far from approaching mental illness as their major public health problem, and one that requires public health thinking and methods. For example, prevention is almost unheard of, and the counties that have public health physicians, paid by the state, do not usually have similar coverage for their mentally ill population.

The community mental health centers, begun with the federal funding impetus in the 1960's, have now lost this source of funds. Community funding has become increasingly difficult, and state support is often minimal as it is in Alabama. Yet, without community alternatives to hospitalization it is difficult to imagine major improvements in state hospitals, much less their "disappearance" as envisioned by the National Institute of Mental Health early in the 1960's.

WHERE SHOULD DECISIVE INTERVENTION TAKE PLACE?

As with other civil rights issues, such as school desegregation, the federal courts have stepped in to take responsibility where it has been neglected by the states. As far back as 1960 Dr. Morton Birnbaum, physician and lawyer, had been advocating the idea of a "right to treatment" for all involuntarily committed patients. In 1966, Judge Bazelon decided in the *Rouse v. Cameron* (373 F.2d 451 [D. C. Cir. 1966]) suit that a man criminally committed to St. Elizabeths Hospital for treatment (carrying concealed weapon; not guilty by reason of insanity) was not in fact getting adequate treatment, merely custody. Therefore, since he had been held for 3 years longer than he would have been if he had been held criminally responsible, Judge Bazelon reasoned that for those 3 years he had been detained without due process of the law. Critics of this decision have pointed out that the justification for confinement without treatment was just as lacking in the first year since the patient was confined for the alleged purpose of treatment. Confinement without treatment becomes punishment.

Since the *Rouse v. Cameron* case occurred in the District of Columbia where there was both federal jurisdiction and a statutory basis for the right to treatment, Judge Bazelon's decision was easier and set less of a precedent than Judge Johnson's decision in Alabama. Legal critics point out that the Bazelon decision is a weak authority for the constitutional right to treatment adduced by Judge Johnson.

In the Alabama right-to-treatment case, *Wyatt v. Stickney* (325 F. Supp. 781 [M. D. Ala. 1971]) the issue was not one concerning only criminal commitment but included civil commitment as well. This suit was brought primarily by hospital employees who had been laid off during a budgetary crisis, not by unhappy patients and their lawyers. The patients were added to the suit almost as an afterthought to bolster the employee plaintiffs' contention that if they were laid off adequate treatment could no longer be offered at Bryce Hospital. The federal court rejected the employees' petition for an injunction against their being laid off, but accepted the patients' part of the suit on constitutional grounds. The plaintiff employees took their part of the case to a local court in Tuscaloosa, the site of Bryce Hospital, and readily succeeded in obtaining a restraining order against the Mental Health Department. Some observers concluded this was a local political decision.

At this stage the lawsuit was more clearly an adversary procedure than it later became, when defendants made many important concessions and refused to defend aspects of their case that were indefensible. Plaintiffs, having decided in advance the incompetence of the Department, requested the court to appoint a panel of masters to determine how the Mental Health Department should be operated, especially how Bryce Hospital should be operated and under what standards. This request was deferred by the federal court initially and has since been deferred indefinitely. The defendants were given 6 months to demonstrate that Bryce Hospital under the new organization, i.e., geographic unitization with unit teams responsible for treatment (and with reduced staff), could become a truly therapeutic institution. (The designated 6 months was a figure apparently taken out of context by the court, because the defendants at no time had contended that Bryce could become therapeutically effective within 6 months. Defendants had contended, rather, that under the new unitization system for the delivery of services, the treatment programs available would reach many more people than they formerly had, even before the layoffs.)

Our next report to the court indicated progress in some areas and not in others, and I think made it clear that more time would be required to implement the various changes that we had suggested.

In our first report we set forth definitions of the mission and the functions of Bryce Hospital that would presumably transform it into a therapeutic institution. In addition, we set forth standards for evaluating the effectiveness of these therapeutic functions. At that point in our thinking this was our preferred interpretation of the court request to set standards. We were not promulgating standards of per diem expenditure, staff-to-patient ratio or physical plant standards for three reasons. The first was that we were still unconsciously acquiescing in the traditional poor funding of state institutions; therefore, we wanted to demonstrate that by improved organization and leadership along with the change in philosophy we could provide adequate treatment for patients without a great deal of new money. I now believe that this tactic was a mistake and probably wasted a lot of time. On the other hand, it may have helped stave off the appointment of a panel of masters which seemed to be urgently desired by the opposition primarily for the purpose of discrediting the Board, the Commissioner and the Mental Health Department.

The second reason was our wish to safeguard our freedom to experiment: comparative effectiveness studies could be made among geographic units, some of which employed differing treatment approaches such as token economy, attitude therapy, group therapy, psychotropic drugs, pastoral counseling, vocational-educational training, and so on. Since we did not soberly expect as an outcome of the suit an influx of scarce and highly paid professionals into the state hospitals and since our resident population of dependent adults with poor educational-vocational-social skills might require different types of staff and programs, we did not wish to be restricted to a traditional psychiatric model of treatment. This would have been capitulation to an a priori judgment that the best and most adequate treatment had been found and is well known. Such is not the case, a point that is well argued in the *Burnham v. Department of Public Health of the State of Georgia* (349 F. Supp. 1335 [M. D. Ga. 1972]) case.

The third reason was that we were well aware that some public mental hospitals—for example, the Veterans' Administration Hospital in Tuscaloosa—had gone through periods in which they were adequately funded and staffed, had adequate physical plants, but still remained essentially static, custodial institutions. In other words, we were trying to persuade the court to abandon any preoccupation with standards of effort or expenditure and to concentrate on standards of effectiveness. From the viewpoint of professional honesty and even novelty this remains an excellent position. From the viewpoint of the necessity to employ the power of the federal court to obtain adequate funding for our public institutions it leaves something to be desired.

The position we took was also an outgrowth of a statewide effort to establish evaluation programs among the mental health centers and the hospitals that would evaluate results rather than effort or expenditure. Actually both kinds of standards are needed. The court's later position that we had not presented any standards remains erroneous in my opinion. We simply had not presented enough standards. We were correct in noting that plenty of money and plenty of staff don't necessarily produce therapeutic effectiveness in an institution. The court was correct in pointing out that without a certain bare minimum of staff any respectable degree of therapeutic effectiveness is grossly unlikely. The problem was: What is a minimum adequate staffing pattern? Were it not for the court order which ultimately tried to enforce unlikely numerical standards of staffing, we could have been in the position of demonstrating therapeutic effectiveness through the use of various staffing patterns. Ideally, the effectiveness of the program should decide what kind of staff and how many would be ideal, not advance preconception about effectiveness. There was very little "Szasz" and even less "Goffman" brought forth in this case. The defendants were well-imbued with some of their best ideas but dared not bring them forth for fear of instant dismissal by the conservative-minded Mental Health Board. The testifying experts, contrawise, showed no such diffidence. They freely set forth the conventional wisdom of each profession.

During the course of the summer of 1971 we invited at least 15 well-known experts in psychology, psychiatry, social work, hospital administration, etc., to come to Bryce, help us assess its strengths and weaknesses and to make recommendations. From the outset we adopted a policy of full disclosure as to the content of their reports to us, so that both the court and the plaintiffs were well aware of the findings of our expert consultants. We had several reasons for doing this, as well as for inviting the consultants in the first place. We wanted to get some outside opinions of people longer in the work and more expert than ourselves as to what needed to be done. We naturally hoped to obviate the necessity in the eyes of the court to appoint a panel of masters to tell us how to run our hospitals. The plaintiffs, along with their personal attacks in the press on the Commissioner, the Board and the Department, had tried to represent in their pleadings that the leaders in the Department were ignorant, callous and incompetent. The court, although ruling against the defendants and for the patient-plaintiffs, refrained throughout the case from adopting such a simplistic view of the defendants.

Finally, we also wished to persuade the court that we were just as interested in the rights of patients as was the opposing side, that we had nothing to hide, and that we were acting in good faith. In brief, we were refusing to be the villains that the other side and the adversary system required for staging a courtroom battle over the rights of patients.

We did not succeed in persuading the court to accept our concept of what standards should be. The most telling order of the court made this clear in the fall of 1971, stating that the institutions were still inadequate and that we had still failed to set standards. However, we did succeed in persuading the court that we were acting in good faith and that there was no necessity at that time to appoint a panel of masters.

I believe it had also become apparent over the summer of 1971, by means of our reports to the court to which the plaintiffs had access, that the case had become less and less an adversary procedure. It increasingly appeared that both sides wanted the same thing (with two exceptions: we did not wish to pay plaintiff's counsel a fee of $50,000, nor did we wish for the court to appoint a panel of masters).

To recapitulate, by 1972, the opposing side had not succeeded thus far in establishing the need for a panel of masters, it had not succeeded in discrediting the Commissioner, the Mental Health Board on the Department, and it had not won the case. It now appeared obvious that only the patients could properly win the case and that the Mental Health Department could not win it except at the expense of the patients. At this stage the arch-conservative Board member from Tuscaloosa remarked in an executive committee meeting, "The only way we can win this case is by losing it." The opposition to the changes now desired by both sides, if any such opposition existed, resided in the lethargy of the legislature, the antifederal poses of Governor George Wallace, and the uninvolvement of the public. As Dr. Karl Menninger remarked on one of his trips to Alabama, "If a patient stays more than a few months in the state hospital, there's something wrong with the state legislature."

The question now pressing was how to lose gracefully, or what stance the Department should adopt in replying to the federal court in order to set standards for the operation of our institutions. The following is a resume of our thinking as of January 1972, quoting from a memorandum I sent to defendants' counsel as the Commissioner:

A. What to ask for as minimal standards:
1. The standards set forth by the Joint Commission on Accreditation of Hospitals, both for the physical facility and the staffing patterns. There are now

172 accredited state hospitals for the mentally ill and 105 non-accredited state hospitals in this country. The State of Kentucky which has almost the same population and per capita income as Alabama has four fully accredited hospitals. This raises two questions. If other state hospitals are fully accredited, why should ours not be so? How can we justify asking for less?

2. The opposition will certainly ask for at least the standards of the Joint Commission, and probably will try for a new set of standards surpassing the latter.

3. If our side should request lower standards or should too vigorously contest the higher standards proposed by the opposition, we would fall into a trap: We were originally accused by the plaintiffs of being complacent in the neglect of patients. Our contesting the setting of higher standards would appear to prove it.

4. If we ask for less than full accreditation we are not only settling for inadequate care for patients, we are choosing to sacrifice large amounts of federal funds, and abandoning the prospect of attracting interns, residents and other high quality professional staff.

B. The question of cost and available state funds:

1. The Administration and the Legislature have proven unresponsive to our budget request. Thirteen million dollars was cut from our $48 million operating budget request and $12 million was cut from our $27 million bond issue request. The latter cut ruled out automatically even minimal renovations at Bryce, Searcy and Partlow.

In retrospect our request was too modest: we followed a course of gradualism expecting excessive reaction from the Governor and the Legislature should we request too much at one session. Therefore, we only asked for enough, $48,000,000, to bring the three institutions' per diem expenditure up to the Southeastern average of $12 a day. The new standards may well cost twice this much.

2. At present the court appears to be our only avenue to adequate funding. Should we try to win the case by arguing that we are doing well enough as is, or with very modest funding, several results appear likely. The first is that we could not win on this basis anyway. If we were to win, it would be at the expense of the patients and we would lose our opportunity to have the strong arm of the court enforcing adequate funding, or alternatively, the release of patients. The latter is not an entirely unreal possibility because the court seems to be preoccupied with the right to treatment as a present right, i.e., one that cannot be postponed indefinitely while we are gradually improving our institutions. I believe the Governor and a majority of our Mental Health Board actually wanted us to take this position, i.e., that we were doing well enough with very modest funding, for various political reasons. However, they did not dare to say openly that they were against full accreditation for our institutions. At one point the Chairman of the Board did make a slip and remark publicly that we could meet the new standards under our present budget. This is manifestly impossible.

Another possible untoward result of our trying to win the case on this shaky basis would be the court's being provoked into ordering a panel of masters to direct our institutions, or even ordering us to pay a $50,000 fee to plaintiffs' counsel!

3. The modest resources of the State are no longer relevant or persuasive. If we were to go on setting standards on that basis, we would once more be acquiescing on the old custom of allowing the Legislature to fund everything else first and human services last.

The court order broadly hinted that judicial funding and/or the forced sale of Mental Health Board lands might be indicated if the legislature did not soon come forth with the necessary funds to finance the new staffing and building standards set by the court.

It is a reasonable estimate that more than 90 percent of the standards set by Judge Johnson at the end of the hearings had already been agreed to by both sides prior to the hearings. Before facing the court hearings the Commissioner and counsel had consulted the Mental Health Board (which governs the Alabama Mental Health Department) as well as the Governor and his advisors. Permission was granted by the Board and the Governor for defendants to submit standards based on those of the American Psychiatric Association, the Joint Commission for Accreditation of Hospitals, and the American Association on Mental Deficiency. Once this was agreed upon with plaintiffs' counsel, nearly all the stipulated standards followed. Later, both the Governor and the Board persistently misinterpreted the stipulations as well as their cost, which we had clearly set forth to them. This wilful confusion formed the basis for the Governor's appealing the case. The Mental Health Board did not follow suit and appeal until it had fired me as the Commissioner.

After all the stipulations, the only standards remaining in dispute were the numerical staffing ratios, about which various expert witnesses expressed widely diverging opinions. There were several difficulties inherent in the minimal staff question: One was few authorities could agree on what that minimum should be. For example, in this case some demanded one psychiatrist for every 10 to 50 patients while others insisted upon one for every 150 or every 250 patients.

Besides, once quality control or standards of output were rejected, one could have only the vaguest idea of what constituted adequate treatment on a statistically demonstrable basis. The court defined "adequate treatment" loosely as one that would offer each patient a reasonable opportunity (according to whom?) for the cure or improvement of his condition. Considering the record of antipsychotic agents since the 1950's and the circumstance that over 80 percent of the patients at Bryce Hospital were being given such medication, a sophist could maintain that the court's definition was being met. That is, he could do so until he discovered that over half the patients at Bryce had been there 5 to 40 years!

In the spring of 1972 the court was confronted with four differing sets of staffing standards: those submitted by the plaintiffs, the defendants, the amici curiae and the Justice Department. The standards offered by the defendants, the most modest of the four, were finally chosen by the court. This was a small victory for the defendants, but they still faced the question of how to obtain enough money to more than double their per diem expenditures. The Governor and the legislature showed no sign of eagerness to provide new funds. (They still have not, being preoccupied with the hope of winning the appeal.) The Mental Health Department had hopes, in the summer of 1972, of being saved by a large infusion of federal funds through the Social Security Amendments. The Department had signed contracts in hand totalling over $150 million by the end of June 1972. The contracts covered in-hospital prerelease programs, transitional services, halfway houses and day treatment programs for most of the patients covered by the order. Shortly after all parties signed the contracts, these federal funds dried up. The Department received less than 10 percent of what had been anticipated.

This was demoralizing: the federal government had one of its courts insisting upon adequate funding as a basis for the right to treatment while the President and Congress defaulted on signed contracts for the federal share of responsibility. It is of some minor interest that Governor Wallace, while appealing the decision of federal judge Frank M. Johnson, Jr., in *Wyatt* did not see fit to appeal this decision, or to sue the Social Security Administration for breach of contract.

Meanwhile, the huge continuing federal subsidies to state highway programs allow and encourage state governments to fund highways first and human services last. This gives federal sanction for an absurd and corrupt order of priorities in the states. Federal grants for hospitals and community mental health centers have been diminishing and are now to disappear. Thus, it would appear that the federal government has almost abandoned all sense of responsibility about the biggest public health problem in the country, at one stroke deserting the hospital patients and the far more numerous outpatients in the community mental health centers.

Even granting the unlikely success of judicial funding (i.e., the court enjoining the legislatures against funding any non-essential service until the state hospital needs were met), the court might rediscover the old adage: "Sue a beggar and catch a louse." Most states do not have enough money to meet the new standards, even if they reorder their priorities in favor of some that are humane and honest. In Alabama, for example, drastic revision of a dishonest and ineffective tax structure would first be necessary. The court cannot order such an obvious step.

The court clearly decided, in the Alabama right-to-treatment case, that the best point of intervention in the long neglect of mental patients was upon the issue of staffing standards and physical plant standards for "a humane physical and psychological environment." The court's insistence upon these standards would then, hopefully, assure adequate funding of the institutions, and adequate staffing would soon follow. The Alabama case has now dragged on almost 4 years and neither of these hopes appears likely to be fulfilled. The legislature of 1973 failed to vote the money for the easy part of the standards: renovation of the buildings. Probably the only move that could force the Governor and the legislature to raise more funds would be for the court to take seriously the "present right" doctrine and order the wholesale release of patients. This might have a stimulating effect on the Governor and the legislature. Besides, fewer than 10 percent of the patients are dangerous.

THE PROBLEMS OF STAFFING

As to the recruitment of professional staff, the experimental evidence shows at least in the short run that advertising and money won't do it. For almost a year before I was fired as Commissioner, the Department advertised in all the leading professional journals and sent recruiting posters to the professional schools. Salaries were described as "open and on the rise," for at that time the staff expected adequate funding through court action or federal money. The results from all this advertising were extremely disappointing. When a trickle of new people did respond, putting their salaries at a new, higher level could and did alienate long-term employees. The latter could not receive raises because of the wage freeze. The federal government again had us in a double bind.

In late September of 1972 the Alabama Mental Health Board fired me as Commissioner and appointed an Associate Commissioner who had been Comptroller to the position. Everything returned to the peaceful stupor of the previous 40 years. The Governor now controlled the newly packed Mental Health Board, who in turn controlled the new Commissioner. New staff appointments showed a comfortable mediocrity. In Alabama this is done by placing "good ole boys" in positions that require experienced professionals. The good ole boys do as they are told. The scarce professionals leave. Recruitment efforts at a national level suddenly lapsed. As if by magic all the torrent of abuse formerly heaped by the press upon the Board and the Commissioner subsided. The Board reversed its position and now sided with the Governor in appealing the case. A sorry spectacle, but perhaps instructive for those who face or will face such suits in their own state hospitals.

As Commissioner I had managed to stay in office 6-months longer than the average tenure for mental health commissioners, which is 3 years and 6 months. It takes 2 or 3 years to learn the job, and both during and after this period of confusion "Time's winged chariot" is indeed hurrying near. One can choose two courses, speed or gradualism. The first involves making enough changes to make enough enemies to ensure being fired fairly soon. One must guess, from the record, that most commissioners have gone this route. Or, one can stay in office longer perhaps by refraining from sudden changes and large decisions and hoping to make changes over the long haul. A handful of commissioners have managed this, to their credit, and it may depend a great deal on personality

In any case, despite a nationwide shortage of psychiatric administrators, commissioners are expendable and replaceable. Indeed, they may all soon be replacing one another in a transcontinental musical chairs game. Just in the past few months half a dozen mental health commissioners, including some of excellence and of long tenure, have resigned or been forced out one way or another.

Each time such a lawsuit descends upon a commissioner, his board of trustees, if any, and his department, all of the usual stresses will be greatly magnified. Villains must and will be found to be punished for the public, professional and legislative neglect of the past 100 years. Staffing problems will multiply, disloyalties and struggles for power will emerge and both organizations and people will show their flaws and occasionally their strengths.

It should be far more simple for the courts to order and accomplish improved physical plant standards than staffing standards. The reasons for the concentration of psychiatrists in private practice in large urban areas are just as personal and sociological as they are economic. Merely finding the money and offering state service salaries roughly competitive with the income of private practice will not necessarily bring a large migration of practitioners into the state hospitals, be they psychiatrists, psychologists, social workers or physicians. Most mature professionals are already doing what they want to do and living where they prefer to live. It will be easier to enlist the young and impoverished professionals and, of course, the tired and old ones who have customarily staffed our institutions.

It may be that the low level of basic medical staffing in state hospitals is only a special case of the failure of medical education and professional organizations to provide medical care in many places where it is needed. For example, there are more than a hundred towns in Alabama that cannot secure a physician through any inducement. Not long ago a failed bill in the U. S. Senate proposed the posting of Public Health Service physicians in towns where they are needed. This is a serviceable idea and might well be applied to state mental hospitals as having populations critically in need of medical services. Another possibility is the drafting of young physicians for 2 years in such public service as mental hospitals and small towns.

It has become clear that medical care is a national, not a local resource. There is something perennially comical about a state-supported medical school clamoring for funds to train physicians for the growing local needs of the state when in fact the majority of their graduates may well become gypsies during their training and settle elsewhere anyway.

In the opinion of some, the concern for medical and nursing coverage in mental hospitals is inappropriate anyway: very few state hospital patients are physically ill. They might well be better served in that aspect of care by a system analogous to "sick call" in the armed services. The hospitals could pay high fees for a few active, competent physicians to provide this service on a contract basis. This arrangement might well be more sensible and economical than providing housing, salaries and fringe benefits to foreign-trained, retired and semi-invalid staff physicians. As to the idea of a great need for numerous psychiatrists in the state hospitals, this too is open to question. Often it springs from the assumption that the population residing in state hospitals is comparable to and needs about the same repertoire of treatment approaches as that of a private mental hospital. This is not the case despite a superficial similarity due to diagnostic labels. A label on a patient in a private hospital mainly means what it says and represents a ticket to what is often honestly considered appropriate treatment. The labels attached to patients in state hospitals are very often mere administrative devices, tickets to inappropriate custody for all sorts of unwanted people. The ticket, or prescription, is written by detached, distant physicians—not by hospital staff. It is made binding by judges, many of whom sign the papers without seeing the patient. Many physicians do the same.

In Alabama, curiously, the counties that send the most "patients" to the state hospitals are usually the same ones sending the most "criminals" to the state prisons. It is often a toss-up, a choice of symptoms or a legal sham, that decides which asylum the aberrant citizen will inhabit. Populations currently hiding out in state hospitals and in state prisons doubtless show important properties in common: low socioeconomic, education and vocational levels; inarticulate patterns of speech; little insight and little inclination to engage in psychotherapy with a typical mental health professional. It has already been demonstrated by numerous community mental health centers that such patients are most effectively helped by "indigenous workers" or "neighborhood people" of similar background. Also, it has become obvious that most people from this segment of society are so weighed down by real survival problems and by their coping deficits due to inadequate social, educational and vocational skills, that they have little energy or interest to contribute to a conventional psychotherapeutic enterprise. There is, by this logic, no good reason to attempt to offer them the traditional prestigious array of professional services by psychiatrists, psychologists and social workers. Rather, we should attempt to discover what such patients need, what service functions can meet those needs, then define hospital service roles as clusters of functions serving those needs. Last of all should we assign titles and arbitrary salary scales to those roles in the hope that the bigger the title the more problems its holder could solve?

In this sense, the *Wyatt v. Stickney* decision could be a long step backward, and could unintentionally cater to the prestige interests of the medical and mental health professionals, few of whom have any interest in state hospitals anyway. Future decisions in right-to-treatment suits could cultivate the ground broken by the Alabama decision by including some fertile additions. One might be that so long as basic standards for health, physical environment and medical care were being met, each hospital would have the freedom to experiment in providing mental health services by using various kinds of staff, including adult educational specialists, vocational teachers, pastoral counselors, etc. The courts could then insist that a yearly evaluation of effectiveness be part of each program, and that results be compared. Indices of effectiveness can be specified and measured.

Without such an open approach the courts will be assuming advance knowledge of the proper solution to a problem far too complex for an authoritative answer at this point. Such an assumption at present can only be based on self-serving and unproven claims of effectiveness by various disciplines.

POSTSCRIPT TO THE *WYATT V. STICKNEY* DECISION

The cool and reasoned language of Judge Sidney O. Smith, Jr., in his decision on the *Burnham v. Georgia* case (August 4, 1972), is in marked contrast to the impassioned rhetoric of all parties, including the court, in the earlier *Wyatt v. Stickney* case in Alabama. In the latter case it would seem that plaintiffs, defendants, amici and the court were filled with indignation at the current status and past record of neglect of the patients in state mental hospitals and were seeking every possible remedy against the likelihood of continuing neglect by the State of Alabama. In *Burnham,* by contrast, the court was reassured on this question by the recent generous appropriations for mental health in Georgia as well as by the state's new statutes guaranteeing the right to treatment in that state.

Plaintiffs had alleged that defendants, the Department of Public Health, State of Georgia and others, provided constitutionally inadequate diagnosis, care and treatment to plaintiffs and to all others similarly situated. On motion of the defendants to dismiss, the district court held, among other things, that plaintiffs could not maintain the action under civil rights statutes, where plaintiffs failed to demonstrate or sufficiently allege the deprivation of a federally protected right. The motion to dismiss was granted.

On first reading, this appears a shallow judgment, lacking in compassion and commitment to the forgotten rights of patients. A closer scrutiny reveals some hard thinking and some philosophical concerns that appear to have been scarcely considered by the parties or the court in the Johnson decision. Curiously, the more "conservative" Smith decision would seem more likely to safeguard innovation and experimentation in state hospital treatment programs. The precedent-setting Johnson decision attempts to safeguard the patients by ensuring a humane physical and psychological environment and adequate staffing in these institutions, but makes a conservative and a priori judgment about what constitutes adequate staffing and adequate treatment. How will these conflicting approaches to helping mental hospital patients be resolved?

The language of the *Burnham v. Georgia* decision will point the way for future judges, plaintiffs and defendants to support or to attach the right-to-treatment argument. The heart of this decision is in the opinion that since each patient is an individual and

since what is good treatment for one might mean disaster for another, the only feasible way in which the adequacy of treatment could ever be measured is against the needs of a particular patient; under these circumstances, class actions of federal rule were not met . . . in that there would be relatively few questions of law or fact common to members of the alleged class, etc., etc.

The Johnson decision assumes that the situation of state hospital patients is all too common, i.e., neglected, and is appropriate for a class action. This was not strictly true. Plaintiffs and defendants agreed that prior to the suit about 15 percent of the patients at Bryce were getting most of the staff's attention.

Since the Smith decision refused to require the State of Georgia to expend additional revenues for the care of mental patients on the ground that said care is already mandated by state law, one combined effect of the Georgia and Alabama cases might be to persuade other states to forestall future lawsuits by the speedy enactment of enlightened mental health legislation. Judge Smith points out that the Bazelon decision was made possible, i.e., the federal court was enabled to take jurisdiction, through the circumstance that Congress had provided for a statutory right to treatment in an area uniquely under federal rather than state control. He also mentions that "Dr. Birnbaum himself has conceded that while such a right to treatment has been accepted by society it has not been recognized as a federal constitutional right." Besides, the court goes on to say, under Georgia statutes involuntary confinement in a state hospital need not rest upon the exclusive premise that treatment must be afforded. Instead, a person may be hospitalized if he is "mentally ill and is (*a*) likely to injure himself or others if not hospitalized, or (*b*) incapable of caring for his physical health and safety." Clinical experience in a mental health center shows far more commitments on the basis of (*b*) and/or because the patient's family is no longer willing or able to keep him than on the basis of (*a*).

Some lawyers and psychiatrists will object that such language is so loose as to practically guarantee the continuing use of state hospitals as paralegal detention centers where citizens can be confined without due process and duly forgotten. Others will maintain that everyday clinical experience makes this broad approach necessary and that the single criterion of dangerousness to self or others would exclude many helpless people whom we are ethically bound to help even if they see no need for it. Each state has decided, or will decide anew, what position to take; either one is open to abuses and disadvantages.

It is intriguing to find Judge Smith, who seems conservative in some ways, quoting Dr. Thomas Szasz in support of the argument that since "psychiatric treatment" covers "everything that may be done under medical auspices and more," therefore, the court can't possibly determine whether or not patients in mental hospitals receive adequate amounts of it. The court wryly comments that the addition of language such as "adequate" or "constitutionally adequate" to a word of uncertain meaning like "treatment" does not clarify but rather compounds the confusion.

The weakest part of the reasoning in the Smith decision is that "there exist multiple adequate remedies at law available to the plaintiffs on an individual basis." Of course they exist, but how many hospital patients are able to make use of these remedies? However, the court goes on to point out plaintiffs' inconsistency in maintaining that the remedies of habeas corpus, medical malpractice and ordinary tort actions fail to provide adequate remedy in that the wrong sought to be remedied affects the system of care as a whole and not on an individual basis. Plaintiffs were at the same time contending that "each individual patient should have his particular therapy or treatment personalized."

Parenthetically, some remarkable successes in mobilizing and re-socializing long-term patients in Georgia's biggest mental hospital had been achieved in recent years through token economy programs. These were not particularly medical or psychiatric, nor were they very individualized. Perhaps Judge Smith had been advised of this work at Milledgeville.

Many psychiatrists are now saying that psychotherapy is essentially a process of education or reeducation. Some would maintain that an insistence upon individualized treatment in the huge state hospitals would be as utopian as demanding individual tutoring for every child in a high school with several thousand students.

Judge Smith's opinion differs most clearly from that of Judge Johnson in its closing paragraphs. It states "The question of what in detail constitutes 'adequate treatment' is simply not capable of being spelled out as a mathematical formula which could be applied to and would be beneficial for all patients."

This is not exactly what the Johnson decision tried to do since it left to the experts the decision as to what individual treatment might be deemed appropriate. However, it did try to ensure adequate treatment by insisting on a mathematical formula providing so many professionals to so many patients. The intention of this approach is clearly laudable and in the tradition of appealing to the Constitution to expand narrow conceptions of civil rights. It still may be the last best hope of mental patients and their care-givers against what remains in most states as continuing neglect and absurd funding priorities set by federal and state governments.

Even so, in his closing lines Judge Smith expresses a concern that should sober all of us who are anxious to be on the side of the angels in this perplexing issue:

The Court is persuaded that some matters are left for legislative and executive resolution short of federal judicial review. All too often, an instance of judicial over-reach can result in a reduction of government services to a minimal level for fear of subsequent accountability for some innovative beneficial program. The rigidity of the court process can often stifle intelligent experimentation in dealing effectively with social problems, often to the detriment of the very persons for whom the litigation is commenced.

Judicial Action and Social Change

DAVID MECHANIC

David Mechanic's contribution changes our focus from the legal and political issues toward an examination of the right to treatment in relation to other forces in the mental health system. To begin, Professor Mechanic succinctly traces the history of mental institutions as a product of contemporary ideology and treatment pragmatism and then he applies this pragmatic and ideological scrutiny to the right to treatment.

He starts by questioning the long-term effect of the current orientation in mental health which has transformed many welfare hotels and nursing homes into mini-institutions for the mentally ill. Mechanic asks if adequate resources can be obtained to provide treatment and then proceeds to challenge the concept of treatment itself. The chapter presents a series of catalytic ideas from the creation of federally funded and maintained minimum standards for adequate treatment to legal recognition of a patient's right to refuse treatment as a necessary corollary to a right to receive treatment. Professor Mechanic concludes by conceptualizing the right to treatment within the context of the fundamental issues surrounding the social control of deviance through involuntary commitment.

The decision of the United States district court in *Wyatt v. Stickney*, 325 F. Supp. 781 (M. D. Ala. 1971) constitutes the frontier of a continuing battle to insure that the mentally ill will have decent and humane care in public institutions. It maintains (as in some previous decisions) that involuntary commitment for the mentally ill, allegedly for their own protection or treatment, is a form of imprisonment and "preventive detention" if the institutions involved do not provide a humane social environment and a specific treatment regimen. The decision puts public officials on notice that the misuse of involuntary commitment for the mentally ill, for the convenience of the community under the guise of treatment and rehabilitation, is an infringement of constitutional rights.

Persons who have been involved and concerned with the treatment provided in public institutions over the years will applaud those who brought the case to court, the involvement of amici curiae, and the court's decision. Nothing in this discussion can detract from the contribution of this decision to the ideals of decency and justice.

My discussion will consider *Wyatt v. Stickney* within a larger social and historical perspective, and will explore the relevance of such legal challenges for mental health developments. I will examine, in a tentative way, how the movement toward the right to treatment relates to other trends and I will speculate on its possible effects.

Movements in the mental health field have always had a strong ideological thrust, although careful examination of their underpinnings suggests more pragmatism than is generally appreciated. Even a cursory history of mental institutions and a brief examination of social processes affecting the mentally ill indicate that there is no stronger combination than ideology and pragmatism. In early colonial history, when mental illness resulted in dependency not attributable to a flawed moral character, the community assumed responsibility for the maintenance of the mentally ill. But the limitations were clear; no matter how worthy the outsider, he was excluded from care or support, and when he appeared he was escorted to the nearest county line.[1]

During the Jacksonian period there was concern with individualism and the growing stress in society, and conceptions of the origins of mental illness shifted from those based on God's will and individual failings to the turbulence of society itself. Since society was the villain, it had a special responsibility to deal with its victims.[2] Insanity was now viewed as treatable by environmental manipulation, and the insane asylum was seen as a model community, protecting the inmate from the turbulent society outside.

By 1860, 28 of the 33 states had established insane asylums. In the preceding years, there was considerable optimism about treatment as great claims were made about curability, and inaccurate and unreliable statistics were promulgated. Later, the basis of these claims was shattered when it was shown that institutions were counting the same patient as multiple cures each time he was released from the asylum. In retrospect, of course, it is difficult to assess the true effects of these institutions; and, in any case, there was enough diversity among them to suggest that what may have been true of one institution may not have pertained to another. Yet, it is reasonable to suspect that the effects of the institutions and the form of treatment some provided (moral treatment) were quite helpful to patients. As Rothman observes, "Medical superintendents designed their institutions with eighteenth century virtues in mind. They would teach discipline, a sense of limits, and a satisfaction with one's position, and in this way enable patients to withstand the tension and the fluidity of Jacksonian society."[3]

Moral treatment had a variety of precepts that sound strangely familiar today. The object of this care was to provide discipline and regularity to the inmate's life in a humane and considerate fashion. It was to be neither brutal nor indulgent, but was meant to induce tranquility and order. Inactivity was considered sinful, and these asylums kept patients busy with a great variety of tasks. Habits of industry and regularity were to be encouraged, and useful work endeavor was the vehicle through which the regimen was accomplished. Work efforts were viewed as both economical and rehabilitative. There was, of course, a thin line between exploitation of patient labor and healthful activity, but it was one of those useful devices that appeared to serve both the institution and the inmate.

In the better institutions there is reason to believe that moral treatment and the organizational regimens associated with it were modestly effective. The basic ideology, whatever its emphasis on discipline, was humane; and, in its early stages, staffing was reasonable. The relationships reported between patient and staff were sympathetic, and the cause of mental illness was seen as a product of the environment rather than as a consequence of the worthlessness of the patient. But all this changed rapidly with growing industrialization and urbanism in the last half of the 19th and early part of the 20th century. With changes in social structure, tolerance for the chronic patient and alien foreigners (who were well represented among them) decreased substantially. Institutionalism was now a convenient way to cope with deviants of all sorts who were difficult to contain in a rapidly growing and dynamic community. Although legislatures provided for asylums, they were not sufficient to cope with the increasing number of inmates incarcerated. With overcrowding and change in the social characteristics of clientele, an era of custodialism began to emerge. Abuses in these institutions became more prevalent, the social characteristics of persons sent to the institutions were increasingly seen as less desirable, and the persons who had options began to avoid the institutions when ever they could. Thus, **asylums** became warehouses for the hopeless, and impoverished, and persons with little power and discredited social status.

The growth of custodialism was concomitant with growing skepticism concerning the rehabilitative effects of asylums. Yet, the institutions continued to be subsidized and built because they performed important functions for an increasingly industrialized and urbanized society, which was less able than before to tolerate deviance. With the demise of the cult of curability and growing pessimism concerning the intractability of mental disorder, less and less attention was given to the environmental conditions of care. This was justified by a growing feeling that mental disorders were organic and unresponsive to environmental treatment, and was reinforced by the growing number of chronic patients sent to asylums from other types of institutions. Thus, institutions developed techniques to manage masses of patients with limited personnel and facilities and at minimum cost.

The product of these forces was a sense of hopelessness and a need for regimentation and control over patients. How else could a small staff deal with hordes of patients destined to a hopeless future? Legislatures faced other needs, and the clients of the asylums were hardly a group to affect political decisions. The reformers who played an important role in the earlier history of the asylum were pushed out by the growing professionalization of the psychiatric profession.[4] The irony was that the new professionals had so little to offer in their stead.

Although there were outcries from time to time against existing conditions in mental hospitals, the age of custodialism was dominant until very recently. Not only was there little treatment and supportive care for patients, but there was also evidence of physical deprivation, abuse, and a regimented, destructive psychological environment. Whatever attention was available was devoted to new patients. Patients who were resistant to early care were relegated to back wards to waste their lives in idleness and despair. Although exposés of the shocking conditions in mental hospitals created attention and concern, other events soon pushed this awareness to the background, and the majority of the mentally ill made few gains. The most influential of these movements in the early part of this century was the organization of the National Association for Mental Health, initiated by Clifford Beer's autobiographical account of his experiences in a mental hospital. Although this movement had considerable influence, it was largely rooted in middle-class values and concerns[5] and had only a marginal effect on the vast numbers of impoverished mental patients.

Like the mental hygiene movement, many of the other developments in the mental health field had little effect on mental hospital operations. The child guidance movement was largely preventive in orientation and was predicated on the assumption that early treatment of deviance could limit later morbidity. The influence of psychoanalysis and its popularity in the United States directed attention away from the mental hospital and the mass of mentally ill, and drew the professional community largely into therapeutic work with less-incapacitated and better-educated clients.

Sociological studies of the mental hospital in the 1950's demonstrated its character.[6] The public hospitals were organized to allow a limited staff to direct and control the activities of large numbers of patients. Life in the hospital was organized around its maintenance, and patients were used to insure that essential work functions were performed. Particularly effective workers were kept in hospitals, since their useful labor was highly valued, while patients who were more impaired or less effective were left alone as long as they caused no disturbance. The average ward was inactive and apathetic, and if patients were vigorous enough to cause a disturbance, a variety of restraints and controls was readily available. Regardless of whatever feelings the staff might have had, the magnitude of numbers forced a custodial ideology and behavior consistent with it.

But even custodial treatment was expensive and, following the Second World War, it was apparent that state legislatures were troubled by the growing costs of incarceration of large numbers of patients who occupied more than half of the hospital beds in the United States. As sensibilites required that the most brutal aspects of hospital wards be eliminated, money was necessary; and the total number of resident patients was also increasing. The states, therefore, were looking for federal leadership and some relief from what appeared as a growing economic burden.[7] In the middle 1950's the introduction of psychoactive drugs had a dramatic impact on the confidence of personnel to deal with the mentally ill. Since pharmaceutical control was now more possible, the reliance on restraints and seclusion was less necessary, and hospitals began to open their doors. Drugs also facilitated the return of patients to the community, since families and the community could more readily cope with patient behavior.

51

The development of the community mental health movement has received wide attention. In our present captivation with this ideology, however, we neglect certain elements that are of interest to the issue before us, and I shall emphasize these aspects. Although the psychoactive drugs were dramatically effective in alleviating some of the most difficult problems of patient management, there is a tendency to attribute more direct significance to drugs than they really had. There is evidence from particular institutions that the open-door policy and administrative change could be accomplished prior to drug introduction.[8] The availability of drugs probably contributed most importantly by giving hospital personnel and the public at large some confidence that community care was feasible, and drugs provided control over the aspects of behavior that were most frightening and disruptive to the community. Thus, drugs facilitated attitudes that eased radical alterations in administrative policy. Also, by the late 1950's, the thinking about the origins of mental illness had once again shifted significantly. Mental disorder was seen mainly as reactive to social conditions and life environments, and there was growing appreciation that the regimen of the custodial hospital had detrimental effects on social functioning and potentialities for future social adjustment.[9] Moreover, evidence linking social inequality to mental health care[10] had a major impact on a profession and a society that were becoming more and more sensitive about this issue. But what made the community-care movement particularly viable was its parallel direction with the needs of the states to find some way of coping with the growing burden of providing care for the mentally ill and the mentally retarded. The economic motivation of the localities was not a trivial aspect of the entire picture and provided the fuel for what was described as a revolution in psychiatric practice.

Many of the states probably would have settled for major federal support to mental hospitals, but they did not prevail in Washington when the details of federal investment were hammered out. Thus, much of the funds came in the form of community programs and construction grants for mental health centers and, later, in money for staffing. Although states and counties were anxious to obtain what funds they could by turning toward programs of community care, they were much slower in spending dollars to provide necessary services for the mentally ill within the community or for helping families and other institutions that were now taking on the burden that had previously been primarily dealt with in hospitals. The administrative action of returning patients to the community occurred quite rapidly, and the trend of mental patients, resident in mental hospitals, showed a sharp decline. The long and hard process of building adequate community services occurred more slowly, and there is evidence that much is still lacking.

Even a cursory examination of the present state of affairs shows an enormous gap between the ideology and realities of community care. While it has been relatively simple to alter administrative policies to avoid hospitalization and to release hospitalized patients as quickly as possible, the development of an adequate framework of community services to assist the mentally ill or their families has been very slow. As economic pressures have mounted for federal and state governments, as well as for localities, there has been less willingness to invest the resources to meet, even minimally, the needs of patients in the community, and the new neighborhood health centers have frequently avoided the most impaired patients. Disturbed and disabled patients are kept in the community under the banner of community care only to suffer community "institutionalism." Various agencies, each attempting to protect its budget, shift the responsibilities to others, leaving many patients greatly in need, unattended and living under appalling conditions.

It is only now becoming apparent to what extent greatly impaired patients have been "dumped" in the community without adequate financial and social resources. In the big cities—like New York—many impaired patients live with other deviants in "welfare hotels" in disorganized areas where they are frequently intimidated and frightened. With poor community care, these patients frequently experience an exacerbation of symptoms and insecurities and, in view of their limited coping capacities, they face horrendous life problems. Although living situations in smaller communities expose the former patient to less disorganized and frightening conditions, similar problems prevail. In the case of schizophrenic patients, it is recognized that aggressive care is required if they are not to regress; but under most community circumstances, this care is not available and former patients simply become lost in the community.

In directing our attention to the conditions of hospital care, we must keep in mind that the responsibilities for patient care in the community are equally important. The fact that a patient is released to the community in no way lessens the responsibility of mental health authorities to insure that there is adequate provision for care. In putting pressure on hospitals, it is possible to encourage the dumping of patients which, under some conditions, may greatly exacerbate their difficulties. In focusing our attention on improved standards of hospital care, we must keep in mind what the state of community facilities is, or we may be in danger of displacing difficult problems from one context to another.

There is no question that many conditions prevailing in mental hospitals and institutions for the retarded are horrible, and that the standards for involuntary hospitalization are extremely lax. No matter how important it is to improve hospital conditions, this improvement should not serve as an excuse to give less attention to due process in involuntary hospitalization procedures. Similarly, if involuntary hospitalization is enforced only as a last resort—which I believe it should be—then there is a special obligation to insure that impaired persons living in the community have adequate opportunities to receive assistance. An adequate conceptualization of the legal problem must, I believe, give considerable attention to the social difficulties of retaining bizarre and impaired persons within the community.

THE PROBLEM OF STANDARDS AND THE MENTAL HOSPITAL

In *Wyatt v. Stickney* the court held that involuntarily committed patients "unquestionably have a constitutional right to receive such individual treatment as will give each of them a realistic opportunity to be cured or to improve his or her mental condition." (A similar case was decided differently in Georgia. These cases have been consolidated and as of August 1973 were under appeal in the United States Court of Appeals for the Fifth Circuit.) The court found that the defendant's treatment program was deficient because it failed to provide a humane psychological and physical environment and a qualified staff in sufficient numbers to administer adequate treatment and individualized treatment plans. The court concluded that "whatever treatment was provided was grossly deficient and failed to satisfy minimum medical and constitutional standards." After hearing evidence from involved parties and amici curiae, the court proposed detailed standards, which it defined as "medical and constitutional minimums." The judge em-

phasized that "a failure by defendants to comply with this decree cannot
be justified by a lack of operating funds."

There can be no legal (or moral) justification for the State of Alabama's
failing to afford treatment—and adequate treatment from a medical
standpoint—to the several thousand patients who have been civilly committed
to Bryce's for treatment purposes. To deprive any citizen of his or her liberty
upon the altruistic theory that the confinement is for humane therapeutic
reasons and then fail to provide adequate treatment violates the very fundamentals of due process.

The court emphasized that "the unavailability of neither funds, nor staff
and facilities, will justify a default by defendants in the provision of
suitable treatment for the mentally ill."

The major precedent for right to treatment is found in *Rouse v.
Cameron*.[11] Judge David Bazelon, in reviewing various criticisms of his
decision in that case, accepts them as appropriate:

(1) Courts are not as competent as hospitals to make treatment decisions;
(2) The evaluation of standards of adequacy and suitability may be next to
impossible in the present state of psychiatry, where "treatment" means different things to different psychiatrists;
(3) No matter how much compulsory treatment is afforded, compulsory
hospitalization is itself generally based on ill-conceived standards and goals and
ought to be reformed radically or discontinued altogether;
(4) The real problem is one of inadequate resources, which the courts are
helpless to remedy—the question posed is one for the legislature and is a basic
policy judgment involving overall priorities in the allocation of scarce resources.[12]

Before exploring these points, it is useful to consider the larger context
of the right-to-treatment decisions.

It is commonly accepted that right-to-treatment decisions expose
the hypocrisy of commitment procedures and injustice in society. The
guise of care and treatment frequently becomes the justification to
remove disturbing members from the community without due process
and with only the most shabby care. By exposing these processes for
what they really are, it is conceivable that influential members of the
community and legislators have their sense of justice aroused and may
take steps to remedy the situation. Moreover, it is possible that court-set
standards of treatment may at least temporarily make unjust practices
more salient, achieve improvements in particular situations, and indi-

rectly encourage authorities to be less abusive of involuntary procedures because it becomes more costly for the authorities to make use of
them.

The issue in *Wyatt v. Stickney* arises from the fact that the patients
concerned are involuntarily incarcerated for the alleged purpose of
treatment and cure. If civil commitment insured due process and
adequate protection of patients' rights, the right-to-treatment issue
would be a much more minor one and one that could be readily resolved.
Since only a fraction of the patients who are presently civilly committed
would continue to be involuntarily institutionalized, the cost of providing a humane environment would be more limited and, hence, conceivably less painful to the taxpayer and the legislature. What makes right to
treatment a central concept is that mental hospitals—particularly in the
backward states—remain as warehouses for second-class citizens, for
the chronically ill, the aged, the retarded, and a host of other poor
unfortunates. Certainly, a reasonable criterion for attacking the conditions in many of these institutions is the constitutional standard protecting against cruel and unusual punishment. But even if this problem did
not exist, the lack of entitlement to adequate care among the handicapped and needy would present problems that the legal approach by itself
could not cope with.

The need for treatment and care does not diminish by improving the
processes of civil commitment. A great many persons in the population
require medical care and support and, with the increasing trend toward
community care and away from civil commitment, there are growing
numbers of needy mentally ill in the community, functioning at very
low levels and suffering from a variety of personal and social troubles.
Community agencies, including welfare services, face cutbacks and
limited budgets, and make efforts to avoid assuming responsibilities for
the mentally ill. One possible unanticipated consequence of treatment
standards for involuntary patients is a tendency to return the patients to
the community without adequate provision for their care and maintenance.

It is well known that the patients who receive least services in
mental hospitals are the most chronic patients. Frequently, the disturbing behavior for which they were originally hospitalized has not been
evident for some time, and they are viewed as neither a danger to
themselves nor to others. Their residence in hospitals stems from the
difficulties of providing suitable living and maintenance arrangements

within the community, and it is frequently felt that such patients who have adapted to hospital life might find continued hospitalization of greater comfort than the realities that face them in the community. The right-to-treatment decisions do not protect patients who may be returned to the community without adequate resources or minimal comfort and support. These patients may suffer in the community or they may return to institutions as voluntary patients without having the protections of the new standards.

Having raised the broader issues, let us consider the specific points referred to by Judge Bazelon. Although I do not believe, in the long run, that court standards can insure appropriate treatment and care, they draw attention to the enormous gap between the legal forms and the realities. As such, they constitute part of the consciousness necessary for social reform.

THE PROBLEM OF INADEQUATE RESOURCES

The standards ordered by the court in Alabama require what, in effect, is a redistribution of benefits among its citizens. This can be appreciated by examining the minimum staffing ratios established by the court: that there be 28 physicians, 48 registered nurses, eight psychologists with graduate training, and 28 social workers per 1,000 patients. However, the state of Alabama had 2,827 nonfederal physicians in 1970, 5,685 registered nurses employed in nursing in 1966, and 65 psychologists—only 39 of whom were clinical—in 1968.[13] The doctor-to-patient ratio in Alabama has been one of the lowest in the nation, approximately 75 to 80 physicians for every 100,000 patients. Even if we assumed that the mental hospitals could recruit the professional personnel required (a highly dubious assumption), it does not follow that meeting these standards would be the most reasonable allocation of such resources.

Americans have grown to regard access to health care as a right, but many citizens of Alabama receive inadequate medical care or none at all. Many of these patients have treatable diseases that can clearly benefit from prompt medical attention. Is it reasonable, then, to insure the kinds of ratios mandated by the court for mental hospitals when it is dubious that many of the patients concerned are treatable by medical intervention? From more humanistic considerations it may be reasonable to reallocate medical services to mental hospitals if for no other reasons than to ameliorate the degrading conditions that presently prevail. But if, indeed, medical staffing is only one of many ways to improve the conditions of the mentally ill, should a solution that is cost-effective be the one chosen?

The State of Alabama is one of the most deprived areas in the United States, and its social and educational services would be deficient on the basis of national comparisons. The court, in searching for an appropriate standard for treatment, could not reasonably use services for Alabamans generally, since such a comparison would hardly insure meaningful care and treatment. Thus, the court established standards on the basis of evidence from experts and national organizations concerned with the quality of mental health services. The theory underlying these standards is one of advocacy for the mentally ill rather than one based on consideration of how society can put its limited resources to best use. I have not checked the data, but I would not be surprised if one cannot make a similar case for deficiencies in Alabama in educational expenditures, class size, teacher preparation, welfare payments, access to primary medical care, social services, county hospital services, and garbage collection.

Since I believe that a national minimal standard is reasonable, then how do Alabama, Mississippi, and other deprived areas achieve the standard? I maintain that the achievement of such a standard is a federal responsibility, and this implies important modifications in how federal health, education, and welfare programs are funded. Birnbaum[14] has argued that financing for the mentally ill in public institutions could be substantially improved by including such patients under Medicare and Medicaid, and insuring that the funds go to the mental hygiene agencies rather than to general revenues. Mental patients in state hospitals are presently largely excluded from these programs. Whatever the weaknesses of recent legislative proposals for federal assumption of direct responsibility for a guaranteed income program, one of its greatest virtues is its ability to bring all areas of the country up to a uniform minimum standard. Matching programs (the more usual mode of federal financing in the health and welfare service area) inevitably come to favor the areas that have the most progressive programs and are most willing to invest their own resources in such programs. Thus, matching-funds programs frequently favor the rich against the poor and sometimes allow the rich to reallocate expenditures already made to new concerns with the initiation of federal programs. However, as the battle in the United States over welfare reform has illustrated, such shifts in the philosophy of funding threaten a variety of vested interests, including the richer states that can be expected to oppose any program of redistribution that diminishes their share. Thus, a viable program probably requires both an increase in overall benefits and redistribution at the same time.

Matching programs have frequently established minimal guidelines and standards for participation—whether in health, welfare, or education. The history of the relationships between the federal government and the various localities gives one little confidence that the federal government has the will or criteria for participation.[15] Civil rights issues have been the most controversial battleground in the enforcement area, but similar failures are evident in welfare administration, Medicare standards for nursing homes and extended care facilities, housing standards, and the like.

STANDARDS OF ADEQUACY AND SUITABILITY

Assuming that it is appropriate for courts to mandate changes in staffing and other resources and in treatment, the issue remains as to whether it is possible to develop reasonable standards and whether the standards established in *Wyatt v. Stickney* are wise. Conformity with them would surely provide a more humane physical and psychological environment for the patient, but the questions remain whether such standards can be reasonably interpreted and monitored, what their long-term effects on mental health policies and practices are likely to be, and their bearing on the untreatable patient and the patient who wishes to refuse treatment.[16]

Although the court was obviously aware of the uncertainties of treatment for the mentally ill, the right-to-treatment cases are based on the assumption that a technology for cure and rehabilitation exists. Judge Bazelon, both in *Rouse v. Cameron* and in his later writings, was clear about the limitations of psychiatric practice. As he noted, however, " . . . it is nevertheless essential to ensure that the patient confined for treatment receives some form of therapy that a respectable sector of the psychiatric profession regards as appropriate—and receives enough of that therapy to make his confinement more than a mockery."[17] In contrast, Thomas Szasz has maintained that:

> The idea of a "right" to mental treatment is both naive and dangerous. It is naive because it considers the problem of the publicly hospitalized mental patient as a medical one, ignoring its educational, economic, religious and social aspects. It is dangerous because its proposed remedy creates another problem—compulsory mental treatment—for in a context of involuntary confinement the treatment too shall have to be compulsory.[18]

Szasz' view is extreme, but it should alert us to real dangers intrinsic to all involuntary treatment. When the psychiatrist is an agent of a voluntary patient, then whatever the uncertainties of psychiatric ideologies and practices, the relationship is one established at the agreement, convenience, and interests of the parties concerned. Since psychiatric ideologies can justify almost any practice under the rubric of treatment, institutional psychiatry not only has enormous power over the patient but also becomes almost impossible to monitor in any specific sense. The psychiatrist comes to utilize ad hoc theories, which he changes and justifies at his convenience. Moreover, it is no secret that mental hospitals of the kind we are considering attract many incompetent physicians and psychiatrists who frequently lack elementary knowledge and understanding of patients' rights. Not infrequently these hospitals recruit foreign physicians who have difficulty speaking and understanding English and who have no grasp of the cultural assumptions that govern their patients' lives.

In his book, *Prisoners of Psychiatry*,[19] Bruce Ennis describes his participation in *Wyatt v. Stickney* and other mental health litigation as part of a New York City Civil Liberties Project. Throughout his book he dramatically illustrates what is so well known by those who have had any sustained contact with psychiatry—that psychiatric concepts are as fluid and changing as the motivation of the psychiatrist using them. In this light, his hopefulness about the effects of *Wyatt v. Stickney* impresses me as unduly optimistic:

> Those standards, if followed in other states, would cause a revolution in institutional health care services. Under those standards, for example, Willowbrook would have to employ eighty-seven psychologists; it now has five. In order to meet the standards, states would be forced to discharge vast numbers of inappropriately hospitalized patients. Those who remained would live in a

normally furnished homelike environment, retainining all the rights of privacy, communication, and human dignity enjoyed by other citizens. And they would be given individualized programs of treatment, job training, and assistance designed to return them quickly to their communities.[20]

It is not as clear as Ennis would have it that the standards would be enforceable. Moreòver, it is not apparent that those patients who would be forced back in the community would have decent and adequate lives, that even minimal services would be provided for them or to assist those who assumed custody for them, and that privacy and dignity would become the institutional norm. Although one can readily identify with such commendable aspirations, it is sobering to consider another revolutionary change initiated by Judge Bazelon and to ponder its course and outcome.

In 1954 Judge Bazelon, in *Durham v. United States*, declared a new test excluding criminal responsibility in cases where the unlawful act was the product of mental disease or defect. The course of *Durham* case law, in expanding the concept of exculpatory mental illness, eventually came full circle when the court of appeals found:

> As an example of this causual connection or relation, if a person at the time of the commission of the crime is so deranged mentally that he cannot distinguish between right or wrong, or, being able to tell right from wrong, he is unable by virtue of his mental derangement to control his actions, then his act is a product of his mental derangement.

Richard Arens reports in his book *Make Mad the Guilty*,[21] on a project involving litigation applying the *Durham* rule to nonpsychotic conditions. In accounting for the rule's failure, Arens maintains that both psychiatrists and the courts basically destroyed its potential. In particular, psychiatrists at Saint Elizabeths Hospital managed their courtroom testimony so as to send unattractive mentally ill persons to jail rather than to accept them on their already crowded wards. Others saw the new rule as a basic threat to the legal process and the presumption of accountability and did what they could to counteract it. The motivation to widen the insanity plea was based on the assumption that more humane care would be more available under this mechanism than through the criminal process. But it became evident that this attempt to bootleg rehabilitation to persons charged with criminal offenses by exculpating criminal responsibility was too radical for the society to accept at the time.

The right-to-treatment approach is one of many strategies used to circumvent our deplorable rehabilitation system and our more inhumane institutions. Whether such mechanisms can be effective is at best an uncertainty, but whatever hopes they have will depend on the ability of courts and the public to seriously audit and enforce specific standards that improve the lives of individual patients. Thus, the standards and their specification are central.

Although one would anticipate that psychiatrists of any persuasion would have welcomed any effort to improve the deplorable conditions in custodial institutions, it was reasonably clear that establishment psychiatry was not exactly euphoric over *Rouse v. Cameron*. The American Psychiatric Association saw this decision as potentially interfering with the psychiatrist's autonomy; and in issuing its official response on the question of adequacy of treatment, the Council of the APA began by asserting that, "The definition of treatment and the appraisal of its adequacy are matters for medical determination."[22] It later justified prevalent custodial practices as forms of treatment.

> The conceptual contrasting of "treatment" on the one hand with "punishment" on the other sometimes obfuscates more than it clarifies the problem. Some Courts, attorneys, statutes, and judicial formulations reiterate, almost ritualistically, that hospitalization without treatment equates with punishment. This is not precisely the case.
>
> Involuntary hospitalization clearly does imply restraint and may be properly viewed as a kind of punishment in a simple, unqualified context. But if such hospitalization is part of a treatment program aimed at interrupting a disease process (even though the treatment is refused or failed), it is not useful to dub it punishment any more than it would be useful to view depriving an addict of the narcotic of his choice as punishment. The utilization of this kind of involuntary restraint may be viewed in one sense as analogous to problems encountered in child rearing wherein there are no sharp delineations as between guidance and discipline or between discipline and punishment, all of which are directed towards putting internal and external limitations on unacceptable behavior. Restraints may be imposed from within by reinforcing a patient's inner defenses, or from without by pharmacological means or by locking the door of a ward. Either imposition may be a legitimate component of a treatment program. Only if the patient were restrained and did not receive any of the treatments cited above could the restraint properly be called punishment. Furthermore, it is unsound to dismiss a procedure as "purely custodial" or "purely punishing" without assessing the total circumstances in which it has been prescribed. The procedure is often of therapeutic value.[23]

As the statement of the Council makes clear, almost any practice seen by some authority in the interest of the patient becomes treatment by definition, and there is very little that cannot be so justified. Erving Goffman's classic descriptions of these processes are even more relevant today than they were when he made them, because institutional psychiatry has increased the sophistication of the theories by which it justifies control practices under the guise of medical treatment.

Regimentation may be defined as a framework of therapeutic regularity designed to allay insecurity; forced social mixing with a multitude of heterogeneous, displeased fellow inmates may be described as an opportunity to learn that there are others who are worse off. . . . The punishment of being sent to a worse ward is described as transferring a patient to a ward whose arrangements he can cope with, and the isolation cell or "hole" is described as a place where the patient will be able to feel comfortable with his inability to handle his acting out impulses. Making a ward quiet at night through the forced taking of drugs, which permits reduced night staffing, is called medication or sedative treatment. . . . Reward for good behavior by progressively increasing rights to attend socials may be described as psychiatric control over the dosage and timing of social exposure. . . . Some of the verbal translations found in mental hospitals represent not so much medical terms for disciplinary practices as a disciplinary use of medical practices.[24]

In light of the above considerations, it becomes essential to consider what standards are reasonably enforceable, prudent, and effective. In general, standards referring to a humane physical and social environment are more amenable to court action than those pertaining to individualized treatment regimens. Of the various standards, those relating to staff-patient ratios, physical standards of the institution, and care of the person are most easily specified and enforced.

There is a growing feeling in the health services field that rigid assignment of functions and restrictions on the efforts of nonprofessionals hamper effective and efficient delivery of health services. The standards, as specified, tend to reinforce existing stratification of work in "psychiatric" tasks and conceivably can have the effect of bureaucratizing treatment and hampering innovation relative to alternative standards. Although the use of the concept of "qualified mental health professional" guards against a medical monopoly, the conditions for allocating "professional" functions to nonprofessionals appear somewhat restrictive. Although I am fully aware of the abuses that this is meant to guard against, I am similarly cognizant of how difficult it will be to achieve the mandated staffing ratios, and an effective program will require the innovative use of nonprofessional staff members.

In *Wyatt v. Stickney* the court also developed specific and enforceable standards concerning physical facilities and amenities. These standards, applied seriously to many state institutions, would require considerable expenditure for rebuilding and remodeling. It is not fully clear what the costs would really be or whether such expenditures, relative to other investments for the mentally ill, would be to their utmost benefit. It is conceivable that such investments, if made, might solidify unwillingness to abandon dependence on such facilities relative to alternate community facilities. Assuming that the application of all new standards involves a specified expenditure of some magnitude, is it not reasonable to have the state reconsider its entire system of mental health care and the alternative levels of care and treatment necessary for a satisfactory program? Standards imposed on one aspect of the system may result in disproportionate resources allocated to mental hospitals relative to newly emerging models of community facilities. Whether the court has any authority beyond the involuntary patient is not clear, but certainly in the case of the retarded population, consideration of alternate facilities would appear to be a reasonable course to encourage.

The difficulty with standards that pertain to actions that are undefinable is that it becomes hard to establish whether the institution is conforming. Often, the conscientious professional will make an effort to meet the spirit of the requirement, and the requirement may interfere with optimal application of his efforts; while the less conscientious professional easily subverts the rule. Having spent a fair amount of time on psychiatric units both good and bad, I am still at a loss to understand how a court will determine that medication is not used as punishment or for the convenience of staff, or that it is unnecessary or excessive. Such standards probably can guard against the most blatant abuses, but they are probably not very useful in regulating more usual excesses.

It is generally maintained that the establishment of an individualized treatment plan is the basis for a rational and humane therapeutic approach. It implies the consideration of the patient's needs, an examination of alternative approaches to meeting them, and it insures a certain degree of planning for each patient. In principle, the establishment of such a program and its continuing review are an essential mechanism; in reality, it can become a farcical ritual that has little to do with the daily conditions affecting the patient and, indeed, its staffing is limited, it may reallocate whatever staff time is available away from contact with patients. It is quite conceivable that professionals come to spend all of their time formulating and reviewing paper plans, while nonprofessional staff continue to run the institution and to have almost exclusive contact with patients. One has only to review the present practice of many institutional psychiatrists to become aware of the large proportion of their time spent on administrative and legal matters. As the staff come to view certain activities as rituals, they sometimes begin rejecting particular patients who by law require certain services. For example, many state hospitals are required to perform physical examinations on newly admitted patients with each admission. Since this is a time-consuming task, medical personnel find patient recidivists (such as alcoholics) a nuisance. To cope with such patients, the staff begin to develop special release and admission policies for them to limit unnecessary work. The long-term consequences of such adaptations may be more dysfunctional than abandoning specific requirements that have their own rationale.

The standards mandated by the court appear to require considerable documentation and review of treatment and control measures. One develops the impression that much professional time would be spent on maintaining proper records that can be useful in court reviews of hospital behavior. But the various standards—no matter how commendable they seem to be—tend to work against one another. We begin with the premise that patients require more attention from mental health professionals. We realize that they are difficult to recruit and are unlikely to be drawn to mental hospital practice, but we forbid one of the major recruiting devices by specifying that all such professionals "shall meet all licensing and certification requirements . . . for persons engaged in private practice of the same profession. . . ." We then specify that those recruited will be required to spend much of their time making entries in records. Each of these requirements, by itself, in a context of adequate recruitment and staff would be reasonable. But are we any better off if we set standards so high that we insure that the institution cannot possibly meet them?[25] If we start by assuming a condition of scarcity and consider how one might use available resources and staff most creatively and effectively, it is likely that we would develop a somewhat different set of standards.

THE COMPETENCY OF COURTS AND
TREATMENT DECISIONS

I do not believe that anyone seriously advocates that courts should make treatment decisions, and thus I find this issue a false one. To the extent that rules are carefully specified so that judgments are possible, I assume that courts can be an appropriate vehicle for reviewing contested judgments by hearing from relevant experts on the issue of appropriateness of care. Courts appear to undertake similar functions in areas equally complicated,[26] and the notion that courts have no business reviewing the contested behavior of physicians is one to which I do not adhere.

Indeed, my experience in the mental health field has convinced me that one of the major difficulties in protecting patients is the awe that many judges have for physicians and the lack of confidence they appear to have in their own judgment. Courts frequently have allowed physicians to make judgments that should be the province of the court, because the judge was unwilling to consider whether the determination required was properly a medical judgment. The abuses of civil commitment are attributable partly to the failure of courts to seriously hear the evidence and their tendency to accept whatever medical advice is given to them. Questions such as "competence to stand trial," "dangerousness," "legal insanity," and the like, frequently have not been examined as social issues involving considerations beyond medical ones. Such decisions are properly community decisions that take into account medical knowledge and behavioral research but involve other considerations as well. Instead, courts have frequently accepted unexamined and unreliable assertions often reflecting little more than personal bias as medical truth and as a basis for decision-making.

In my view, courts must develop more competence in making judgments concerning mental illness on the basis of the facts with greater awareness of the appropriate bounds and limits of medical and psychiatric evidence. The willingness to blandly accept such evidence and to shift responsibility from the court to the physician has caused much injustice. I can think of no greater contribution the courts can make to the involuntary patient than to take their claims seriously and to give them their day in court with full due process.

One of the issues left unresolved by the court in its standards in *Wyatt v. Stickney* was the case of patients who wish to refuse treatment, and I am not convinced that in this area the judge made the most appropriate determination. Although the standards specify that "patients have a right to be free from unnecessary or excessive medication," the patient's right to refuse involuntary medication is not protected. Patients are protected against experimental research without consent, against major physical treatments (such as ECT), against adverse reinforcement conditioning, and "other hazardous" treatment. Although patients' rights to be free from physical restraint and isolation are guaranteed except in emergencies, medication is treated as an exception. This exception, therefore, deserves inspection.

Today, drug therapy is the most significant treatment modality available to psychiatry. There is considerable evidence of its usefulness in treating depression and in the maintenance of schizophrenic patients. Medication, however, has been one of the most frequently abused means of ward maintenance and patient control. Although most of the mandated standards are consonant with the viewpoint that mental patients can reasonably exercise judgment in their own behalf, the right to refuse medication—one that is available to almost any other kind of patient—is denied. In my view, this treatment power of the hospital is in conflict with a humane hospital environment. In a busy and active ward the availability of involuntary medication becomes a substitute for the time-consuming efforts to achieve voluntary consent through persuasion and trust. I am not maintaining that extending this right would not create some problems, as do many of the other mandated standards: there may be occasions where involuntary medication is justified and sensible. But one must consider both the benefits and costs, and I believe that the extension of the right to the patient to refuse medication would do more to insure his integrity than almost any other standard.

The dilemma of the patient who refuses treatment exists only in respect to the standards relevant to individualized treatment programs. Certainly such patients, regardless of what course they choose, would benefit by improved physical conditions, the protection of their rights, and a more humane physical, psychological, and social environment. A prudent application of the right-to-treatment standard should require no more than that the hospital unit on which the patient resides have sufficient facilities, staff, and treatment modalities to provide a minimal acceptable standard of care. In my view, all that a unit would have to demonstrate to meet this requirement is that facilities are available and that a reasonable effort was made to extend them to the person involved. It would be unfortunate, indeed, if the right to treatment became a new form of tyranny that limited the patient's options.

The above position presents some problems relative to the patient who refuses treatment but who finds the new hospital environment a comfortable and attractive place. There is evidence that, for some patients with long-term chronic disabilities who face difficult and impoverished community conditions, a decent hospital environment can become a refuge from the outside world.[27] To the extent that such patients are involuntary and are extended the right to refuse treatment, there are few options. Under some conditions such involuntary patients can be released and be readmitted voluntarily, contingent on their acceptance of certain types of treatment. For patients who cannot be released, we may have to accept their lack of cooperation as the price society must pay for continuing to depend on involuntary commitment procedures. Since this issue is the key to the larger problem, let us examine it.

THE REFORM OF INVOLUNTARY PROCEDURES

In one sense, right to treatment is an indirect attack on the current abuses of involuntary procedures, such as in civil commitment and in incompetency to stand trial. But in another sense, the right-to-treatment approach encompasses an endorsement of the medical model in contrast to competing views of the conflict between patient and community. Although the right-to-treatment approach attacks commitment procedures where they are perhaps most vulnerable, by exposing how little treatment is made available, there is danger of implicitly accepting the idea that the provision of treatment is the only issue at stake. This approach potentially is harmful if it implies that even superb treatment lessens the obligations of the community to provide rigorous due process in commitment procedures, or if it suggests that the patient is obliged to accept specific treatments for either a limited or prolonged period. If we create the illusion that because the services offered in mental hospitals are appropriate by the standards of "a respectable sector of the psychiatric profession" that there is less need to be vigilant in protecting the civil liberties of the patient, then the right to treatment can become a retrogressive step in the development of a more humane social policy.

Although I belive the intention of right-to-treatment advocates is to fundamentally recast mental hygiene approaches and to maximize patients' dignity, there is always the danger that the community in its incremental approach to social change will adopt the posture, but not the substance, of the position. It is conceivable that, by improving some aspects of hospital care, public officials may deflect criticism of the processes that violate patient rights and inadvertently may help to sustain the existing pattern of removing bizarre and disturbing persons from the community even when they pose no great threat. Let us make no mistake about it; communities will continue to insist that bizarre and annoying members be removed. The pressures for incarceration are considerable, and it is only through concern and vigilence that abuses can be minimized. Also, if community pressures are to be resisted, mental health programs in the community will have to be sophisiticated and attuned to possible difficulties.

The right-to-treatment issue alerts us to a fundamental difficulty— the failure to insure an adequate level of treatment entitlement to citizens as a whole. For if the courts act to protect the treatment rights of the involuntary patient, it is hard to imagine that legislatures will not insist that voluntary patients receive at least comparable services. If successful, then, these suits will create societal dissonance that will contribute to social reforms. The question of how successful such suits can be in the long run is a difficult one. Even small gains are not to be minimized, and in conjunction with other challenges to some institutional psychiatric practices and involuntary care, real improvements are possible.

Recent litigation in the area of patients' rights, taken as a whole, must be seen as attempts to undermine existing mental hygiene legislation and its role in society. Bruce Ennis has stated the matter quite candidly, "So much is wrong with involuntary hospitalization that a reasonable tightening up of commitment standards and a modest extension of patients' rights would cripple the enterprise beyond recovery."[28] It is not so clear, however, that the courts and the legislatures are prepared to allow such a useful mechanism of social control to suffer such injury. It is more likely that they will attempt to adapt to external attack by modifying the most abusive practices, by providing greater opportunities for review, and by attempting to improve those most visible conditions that arouse public concern. It is essential for those who attack such injustices by litigation to be ambitious but also realistic about possible achievements and dangers. The mental hygiene bureaucracies of the various states have enormous resources and advantages. They can deplete the energies and resources of their antagonists without undergoing fundamental change. Although litigation creates temporary discomfort, it is difficult without constant surveillance to insure that gains achieved can be maintained in the future. Perhaps what worries me most is that in the event new standards can be sustained, hospitals will increasingly unload their less attractive patients to other institutions that are even less humane or release them to the community without decent care and attention. Already there is considerable indication that such practices are being followed under the pressures of funding and under the guise of the new community psychiatry ideology. While it may be true that many hospital patients are not appropriately amenable to civil commitment and would not be commitable if the process had greater integrity, many suffer from significant handicaps that require assistance.[29] I fear that it is not unlikely that they will find themselves back in the community with few benefits and supports, and the new pressures on mental hospitals will make them less willing to accept these patients voluntarily or as part of their community programs. We should not forget the fate of the well-intentioned *Durham* rule.

The existing conditions in our institutions and procedures for handling persons who violate community norms are deplorable. However, it is not evident that the litigation approach, by itself, can have a lasting effect. A just and effective rehabilitation system must exist within a larger context of justice for the deviant, the impoverished, the disenfranchised, and the sick; and there must be a greater understanding of how to deal more effectively and equitably with such persons. No matter how astute the litigants or how passionate the court, the long-term quality of our hospitals, our rehabilitation institutions, our schools, and our society generally depends on more fundamental decisions made through the legislative process. The fact that litigation may arouse the conscience of the legislature and the concern of the public is evident. But in the long haul, the fate of the mentally ill, like all other unfortunates, is in the hands of the people who make and administer the laws and the persons who elected them. It seems, then, that the rights of the mentally ill must ride the crest of other waves that entitle all citizens to certain benefits to enhance and protect their health. These benefits should be considered as property[30] to be used on one's own volition.

NOTES

1. A. Deutsch, *The Mentally Ill in America* (New York: Columbia University Press, 1949), p. 45.

2. D. Rothman, *The Discovery of the Asylum: Social Order and Disorder in the New Republic* (Boston: Little, Brown, 1971), pp. 109-29.

3. *Ibid.,* p. 154.

4. G. Grob, *The State and the Mentally Ill* (Chapel Hill, N.C.: University of North Carolina Press, 1966).

5. K. Davis, "Mental Hygiene and the Class Structure," *Psychiatry, 1* (1938), 55-65.

6. I. Belknap, *Human Problems of a State Mental Hospital* (New York: McGraw-Hill, 1956). and E. Goffman, *Asylums: Essays on the Social Situation of Mental Patients and Other Inmates* (New York: Doubleday-Anchor, 1961).

7. D. Mechanic, *Mental Health and Social Policy* (Englewood Cliffs, N.J.: Prentice-Hall, 1969), pp. 57-61.

8. D. Mechanic, *Medical Sociology* (New York: Free Press, 1968), pp. 383-85.

9. Joint Commission on Mental Illness and Health, *Action for Mental Health* (New York: Science Editions, 1961).

10. A. Hollingshead, and F. Redlich, *Social Class and Mental Illness* (New York: Wiley, 1958).

11. 373 F. 2d 451 (D. C. Cir. 1966).

12. D. Bazelon, in D. Burris (ed.), *The Right to Treatment* (New York: Springer, 1969).

13. National Center for Health Statistics, *Health Resources Statistics—1970.* Public Health Service Publication 1509: 134, 153, 198 (Washington, D.C.: U.S. Government Printing Office, 1971).

14. M. Birnbaum, "The Right to Treatment—Some Comments on Implementation," *Duquesne Law Review, 10* (1972), 578-608.

15. J. Handler, *Reforming the Poor: Welfare Policy, Federalism, and Morality* (New York: Basic Books, 1972).

16. J. Katz, "The Right to Treatment—An Enchanting Legal Fiction?" *University of Chicago Law Review, 36* (1969), 755-83.

17. Bazelon, *op. cit.,* p. 2.

18. T. Szasz, "The Right to Health," in D. Burris (ed.), *The Right to Treatment* (New York: Springer, 1969).

19. B. Ennis, *Prisoners of Psychiatry* (New York: Harcourt Brace Jovanovich, 1972).

20. *Ibid.,* p. 108.

21. R. Arens *Make Mad the Guilty: The Insanity Defense in the District of Columbia* (Springfield, Ill.: Thomas, 1969).

22. Council of the American Psychiatric Association, "Position Paper on the Question of Adequacy of Treatment," *American Journal of Psychiatry, 123* (1967), 1458.

23. *Ibid.*

24. Goffman, *op. cit.,* pp. 380-82.

25. See L. Friedman, *Government and Slum Housing: A Century of Frustration* (Chicago: Rand McNally, 1968).

26. D. Bazelon "Implementing the Right to Treatment," *University of Chicago Law Review, 36* (1969), 742-54.

27. A. Ludwig, *Treating the Treatment Failures;* The Challenge of Chronic Schizophrenia (New York: Grune and Stratton, 1971).

28. Ennis, *op. cit.,* p. 230.

29. B. Pasamanick, F. R. Scarpitti, and S. Dinitz, *Schizophrenics in the Community* (New York: Appleton-Century-Crofts, 1967); G. W. Brown, et al., *Schizophrenia and Social Care* (London: Oxford University Press, 1966); and A. Davis, et al., "The Prevention of Hospitalization in Schizophrenia: Five Years After an Experimental Program," *American Journal of Orthopsychiatry, 42* (1972), 375-88.

30. C. Reich "The New Property," *Yale Law Journal, 73* (1964), 778-87.

EDITORS' NOTE: This chapter originally appeared in *Politics, Medicine and Social Science* (New York: Wiley-Interscience, 1974).

The Right to Habilitation: Litigation as a Strategy for Social Change

CHARLES R. HALPERN

Until the *Wyatt* decision, the concept of right to treatment was only applied to mental illness. In the next chapter, Mr. Halpern focuses discussion on the rights of the mentally retarded to receive treatment. The chapter begins with a description of the historical and legal development of the right to habilitation for the mentally retarded. Mr. Halpern, who was one of the principal attorneys in the *Wyatt* case, analyzes both the strengths and limitations of litigation as a strategy for social change. Although the *Wyatt* case has stimulated other litigation as well as legislative reform, he notes that the ultimate impact of right-to-treatment cases depends upon continued public awareness and political action. In conclusion, Mr. Halpern views the adequacy of community services, sterilization of the retarded, and the right to refuse treatment as several unresolved issues that have emerged from the right to habilitation.

The legal system, in the past, has shown little interest in the problems of the mentally ill and mentally retarded. The system provided an expeditious process for expelling such people from society and a conceptual justification for keeping them out of sight and far away. Once they had been placed in institutions, the courts' interest was at an end. Mentally ill or retarded people did not lose their citizenship when they entered the institution, but the courts' lack of interest, combined with the unavailability of legal representation, left the people in the institutions in a legal limbo. They were citizens, protected by the Constitution, but their rights existed only at the sufferance of the professionals and custodial personnel hired by the state to look after them. And their complaints of infringement of rights were discounted because they were regarded as unreliable witnesses to their own situation.

Predictably, conditions in the institutions that housed the mentally impaired were grossly inadequate. Periodically, a burst of reformist zeal would publicize the abominable conditions that often existed in these institutions; but such episodes were spaced infrequently, and they rarely led to genuine institutional reform.

In this chapter I shall focus on the recent development of a new concern in the legal community with the rights of the mentally impaired in institutions. Within the past 10 years, courts and lawyers have begun to define the constitutional protections that follow mentally impaired people into such institutions. Statutes passed to protect these groups, which had been largely ignored, are being taken seriously; courts are beginning to demand that good legislative intentions be matched with adequate performance. A small but significant group of lawyers is undertaking to provide representation to mentally impaired institutional residents. Perhaps the most significant dimension of this new legal interest is its insistence that mentally impaired people be treated as *citizens*.

The "right to treatment" is a shorthand reference for the rights of mentally impaired people in institutions. For the mentally retarded, who are not "sick" and in need of "treatment," the term "right to habilitation" has come to be used. In this chapter, I shall emphasize the legal rights of the mentally retarded and the right to habilitation. I shall discuss at some length the case of *Wyatt v. Stickney*,[1] and consider some of the legal problems which right-to-habilitation litigation has brought to the surface.

The judicial process will not quickly or easily bring justice to the mentally retarded. The systematic exclusion and degradation of the retarded has been a *de facto* national policy which satisfies deeply felt needs—for example, the need to exclude people whose behavior is incomprehensible and, therefore, threatening; and the need to affirm the primacy of intellect and reason by demeaning those who are deficient in these qualities. Moreover, it has been relatively cheap and easy. Our policies have led to the building of massive institutions and the creation of entrenched bureaucracies that are extremely resistant to change. A few lawyers representing the interests of the retarded and a few judicial decrees cannot change these basic realities overnight. But the legal system can undo some of the mischief it has created. It can interpose constitutional limitations on the ways society and professionals deal with the mentally retarded. It can make visible presently invisible decisions which degrade the retarded. And it can focus attention on anachronistic practices that reflect antiquated notions of mental retardation and are inconsistent with fundamental concepts of decency and morality. In these ways the legal process can serve as a catalyst in a complex process by which legislatures, professionals, and the public can be brought to seek humane ways of dealing with the retarded, which recognize their capacities as human beings and their rights as citizens.

WAREHOUSES FOR THE RETARDED—
OUR INHERITED INSTITUTIONS AND STATUTES

Any reform movement takes its shape, in part, from the institutions and ideologies that it inherits from the past. To understand the development of the right to habilitation, one must first understand the institutions to which the mentally retarded are consigned and the legal framework that maintains and legitimizes these institutions. The term "right to habilitation,"[2] as usually used, refers to rights in institutions flowing from the Constitution, although it can also include rights defined by statute or administrative regulation. No general right to habilitation for retarded persons living in the community has yet been developed. Thus, even this progressive development in the law mirrors the archaic system of institutionalization that we have inherited.

The fact that reform efforts have focused on the rights of the institutionalized mentally retarded, however, should not lead to acceptance of the legitimacy of institutionalization. It is impossible to discuss a right to habilitation intelligently if it is not recognized that the dichotomy between institution and community, with its implication of permanently isolating the retarded in institutions, is antithetical to adequate habilitation. Judicial intervention which reinforces this inherited dichotomy does not enhance the welfare of the mentally retarded. The best modern thinking in the mental retardation field subscribes to the principle of normalization, a principle which urges that the mentally retarded should live a life style as normal as possible. A corollary of the normalization principle is that the treatment of the mentally retarded in large, barracks-like institutions is inappropriate.

Statutes concerning the mentally retarded purport to define a population which is "feeble minded," "mentally inferior or deficient," or "mentally defective" because it fails to meet some vaguely articulated criterion of intellectual and social competence.[3] The Alabama statute, for example, permits involuntary commitment of a person who "is unable to care for himself, to manage his affairs with ordinary prudence, or is a menace to the happiness or safety of himself or others in the community, and requires care, supervision, and control either for his own protection or for the protection of others."[4]

This representative statute employs vague but absolute terms. It characterizes a class of mentally retarded persons that is unable to survive in the community. The commitment process entails a timeless negative judgment: this is a person who cannot make it on the outside. It recognizes no nuances. Such a simplistic formulation precludes consideration of other questions which should be asked:

> In what setting could habilitation services be most effectively delivered?
> What habilitation program would entail the least interference with the retarded person's freedom?
> What services would permit this person to continue to live in the community?

The statutory scheme does not invite consideration of temporary institutionalization for short-term skills training, designed to return the retarded person to the community with enhanced competence.

The character of the institution to which the mentally retarded person is committed follows from this definition of the institutionalized population. Most of these institutions are hopeless places dedicated to the lifelong custodial care of residents. They are isolated from the larger community, often located in places that are geographically remote from major population centers. They are discrete units, with no outreach and no coordination with the facilties that serve the mentally retarded in the community. They lack a habilitation commitment; indeed, the staff frequently feels that many or all of their residents are beyond habilitation. They are grossly underfunded, often relying on uncompensated resident labor for maintenance. The people who staff such institutions, at professional and nonprofessional levels, do their dreary work without peer approval or public credit. Institutions of this character generate abuse and neglect of residents and cause deterioration of their physical and mental condition. Historically, these conditions have led to cycles of exposure, public outrage, and expressions of reformist enthusiasm, punctuating long periods of public neglect and indifference.

In almost every state, these old style institutions persist, and their mentally retarded residents suffer. The existence of these institutions is increasingly anachronistic. In recent years, attitudes toward mental retardation have changed radically and habilitation techniques have improved. The giant institution set off in a rural community is no longer the preferred model for treating the mentally retarded. Systems that focus on community-based care—on group homes, day care centers, sheltered workshops, family counseling, respite care and the like—can and should replace the older model.

Moreover, it has been recognized that the commitment process does not select only the mentally retarded most desperately in need of institutional care. Such vague criteria of social ineptitude as "inability to manage affairs with ordinary prudence" and "need for care, supervision and control" import a wide range of extraneous considerations which have nothing to do with the mental competence of the person himself. A retarded person in a family that can afford private nursing aid is less likely to be institutionalized than a retarded person from a poor background. A person who has the good fortune to live in a place where supportive services for the mentally retarded are available in the community is less likely to be institutionalized than one who lives in a place without such community facilities. And the presence of physical defects in addition to mental defects can often be a dispositive factor. Indeed, since many persons are committed to institutions in their infancy, the educational background and ideology of a retarded child's pediatrician is likely to be a major factor in the determination of whether he should be institutionalized. Furthermore, the heterogeneity of the institutional population is increased by the commitment of mildly retarded people who are institutionalized because it is thought that their antisocial behavior is more humanely dealt with through an institution for the retarded than through the criminal system.

The mentally retarded are a diverse group, with widely varying capacities. The range of habilitation services they need is equally varied. yet, the institutional and legal framework fails to recognize this diversity. The dilemma of the lawyer trying to establish and implement the constitutional rights of the institutional resident is to pursue this objective without adding to the legitimacy of the institution. In pursuing this objective, efforts to remedy institutional abuses must be paired with efforts to develop a full range of alternative, community-based services, such as adequate educational opportunities, less restrictive residential settings, and support services that will assist the retarded in independent living.

Many retarded persons now institutionalized should not be in institutions at all; they should be living in the community. It would be a misfortune if the net impact of right-to-habilitation litigation was to generate a misguided effort to turn massive institutions, which are beyond redemption, into suitable habilitation settings. Such institutions by their very nature—their size, their isolation, their impersonality, their tradition—are unsuitable for habilitation.

THE ELEMENTS IN THE LITIGATION REVIVAL

The current legal efforts to improve the condition of the mentally retarded involve several complementary strands. First, citizen groups, like the National Association for Retarded Citizens, and professional groups like the American Association on Mental Deficiency, are joining with concerned attorneys to improve the systems that deliver services to the retarded. Second, there is a general disillusionment with incarceration as an all-purpose response to deviant behavior; this applies to juveniles, mental patients, and prisoners as well as to the retarded. The adverse consequences of institutionalization itself have been studied and documented.[5] Third, lawyers working in poverty law offices, civil liberties projects and public interest law firms, are turning their attention to the rights of the mentally impaired. Fourth, the development of new mind-changing techniques—including psychoactive drugs and behavior modification—together with their expansion into nonmental health institutions such as schools and prisons, has created some uneasiness about professionals backed by the force of the law, who purport to define normal behavior and make people conform to their norms. Finally, in the case of the retarded, there is a growing recognition that retardation is not a static, hopeless condition; but rather, retarded people have a developmental potential that has been disregarded in the past.

It is impossible to state precisely how these factors interrelated in bringing about the recent attention to the problems of the mentally impaired within the legal system. But, when these problems were brought to the courts, it is not surprising that they found receptive forums. At least since 1954, the date of the Supreme Court's decision in *Brown v. Board of Education,*[6] the federal judiciary has shown a special concern with the constitutional rights of minority groups that are incapable of asserting their interests through the political process. More particularly, in recent years the courts have begun to delineate the constitutional rights of those confined in total institutions—jails, prisons, mental hospitals, and juvenile detention facilities.

DOCTRINAL BASES FOR THE RIGHT TO HABILITATION

A variety of constitutional arguments have been made to establish the right to habilitation. The Constitution itself, of course, does not explicitly prescribe a right to habilitation. The right follows as a corollary from the guarantees of due process and equal protection, and from the constitutional prohibition of cruel and unusual punishment.[7]

Civil commitment deprives a mentally retarded citizen of his personal liberty, an "interest of transcending value,"[8] on which other constitutionally protected rights depend. Civil commitment is one of those exceptional processes by which the government can incarcerate a person who has committed no crime, without rigid adherence to constitutionally prescribed procedures. Such processes are closely scrutinized by the courts.[9]

Involuntary commitment to an institution for the mentally retarded is indisputably confinement of a most onerous kind. Benevolent motivation for such confinement is overwhelmed by a harsh reality. The person confined is taken from his normal surroundings and placed in a massive, isolated, prison-like institution. The details of his life are regulated by an impersonal bureaucracy, and he is stripped of his individuality and privacy.[10] For retarded persons who have considerable autonomy before commitment, the deprivation is great. For others, who have relatively little autonomy because of the severity of their retardation and physical impairments, the deprivation attendant upon institutionalization will be relatively less severe. Nonetheless, the isolation from family and familiar surroundings, and the subjection to institutional routines and a barren environment constitute a deprivation.[11]

Due Process

The Supreme Court has stated that involuntary confinement of the mentally impaired must be measured by a due process yardstick. In *Jackson v. Indiana*[12] a mentally retarded man who was deaf and could not speak was found incompetent to stand trial and confined to a mental institution. He was not provided with suitable habilitation or programs calculated to make him competent. The Court held that his confinement for a period of three and one-half years under those circumstances violated his right to due process of law. The unanimous Court, speaking through Mr. Justice Blackmun, said: "At least, due process requires that the nature and duration of commitment bear some reasonable relation to the purpose for which the individual is committed."[13]

Under the *Jackson* decision, the due process clause imposes substantive requirements on the "nature" of confinement; there must be a "reasonable relation" between the nature of confinement and its purpose. Since statutes for the confinement of the mentally retarded are statutes intended to assure adequate habilitation, any confinement without habilitation under this theory violates due process. Habilitation is a necessary element for any constitutionally acceptable scheme for the civil commitment of the mentally impaired. As the *Wyatt* court stated: "Adequate and effective treatment is constitutionally required because, absent treatment, the hospital is transformed 'into a penitentiary where one could be held indefinitely for no convicted offense.' "[14]

Cruel and Unusual Punishment

The nature of confinement in institutions for the mentally retarded must be measured against the eighth amendment prescription of cruel and unusual punishment, notwithstanding that the mentally retarded person is not confined for punitive purposes.[15] While confinement reflects a humanitarian intention to assure adequate habilitation, the fact remains that "any deprivation of liberty, incarceration, or physical detention is, in reality, a form of punishment."[16] Hence, the nature of confinement of the mentally impaired must be reviewed by the courts under the eighth amendment standard.[17]

The cruel and unusual punishment prohibition is not limited to physical torture or barbaric mistreatment; judicial interpretation has broadened the concept. Imprisonment of a narcotics addict for 90 days without treatment has, for example, been held by the Supreme Court to constitute cruel and unusual punishment.[18] In *Robinson v. California,* the court held that drug addiction and that punishment for an illness is unconstitutional; and confinement for compulsory treatment would, however, not violate the eighth amendment:

It is unlikely that any State at this moment in history would attempt to make it a criminal offense for a person to be mentally ill, or a leper, or to be afflicted with a venereal disease. A State might require . . . that the victims of these and other human afflictions be dealt with by compulsory treatment, involving quarantine, confinement, or sequestration. But, in the light of contemporary human knowledge, a law which made a criminal offense of such a disease would doubtless be universally thought to be an infliction of cruel and unusual punishment in violation of the Eighth and Fourteenth Amendments.[19]

Under the reasoning of the Court in *Robinson,* incarceration of mentally retarded persons without adequate habilitation violates the eighth amendment ban on cruel and unusual punishment. Mentally retarded citizens suffer from an impairment that requires specialized habilitation. Confinement without such habilitation is indistinguishable from penal confinement.

There is another sense in which the cruel and unusual punishment prohibition of the eighth amendment is relevant to the institutionalized mentally retarded person. Regrettably, conditions in many institutions are so substandard that confinement of the mentally retarded in them violates basic norms of decency. For example, conditions shown to exist in the *Wyatt* hearing—the physical deprivation, the lack of basic sanitation, the overcrowding, the lack of physical exercise, the inadequate diet, the unchecked violence of residents against each other and of employees against residents, the lack of adequate medical and psychiatric care, the abuse of solitary confinement and restraint—constitute cruel and unusual punishment. Indeed, the conditions bear a close resemblance to conditions that have been held to constitute cruel and unusual punishment in cases involving convicted criminals and persons accused of crimes.[21] A fortiori, these conditions subject the mentally retarded residents to cruel and unusual punishment.

Equal Protection of the Laws

The equal protection clause of the fourteenth amendment requires scrutiny of the standards by which persons are classified by law. The guarantee insures that a minimal standard of equity and reasonableness constrains the process by which government regulation allocates burdens and benefits. Where fundamental rights are affected, the courts will scrutinize classifications closely. In such cases, the classification must be "measured by a strict equal protection test" and the government has the burden of showing "a substantial and compelling reason" for the classification in question.[22]

Classification of retarded citizens for purposes of institutionalization affects the most fundamental rights of the persons committed.[23] It involves massive abridgement of the right to liberty and necessarily infringes on other fundamental rights, including the right to travel and the right of free association.[24]

Commitment statutes typically define mentally retarded people as a class that is in need of some kind of special habilitation service.[25] The basis for the classification of persons to be committed and the characteristic that sets the members of that class apart from the rest of the population is the fact that each of them suffers from a degree of mental impairment which requires that special habilitation be provided. (The mere fact that such persons are socially inept or incapable of looking out for their own welfare would not justify such classification and confinement. States have no general policy of providing involuntary care in incarcerative settings to socially inept citizens who are not mentally impaired.)

Mental retardation is a constitutionally permissible basis for a classification that affects fundamental rights *only* if the state provides persons in this class with suitable habilitation. As the Supreme Court has held in another context, "equal protection does not require that all persons be dealt with identically, but it does require that a distinction made have some relevance to the purpose for which the classification is made."[26] For the mentally retarded people who are committed to institutions, "the purpose for which classification is made" is to provide habilitation. If the mentally retarded are confined without habilitation, "all semblance of rationality of the classification" purportedly based on the need for habilitation disappears.[27]

JUDICIAL RECOGNITION OF THE RIGHT TO HABILITATION

The legal rights of the mentally retarded have been neglected more completely even than the rights of the mentally ill. In the judicial process, mental illness has been at least a matter of marginal interest; mental retardation was a matter of no interest at all. Hence, it is not surprising that the right-to-treatment concept for the mentally ill developed prior to the right-to-habilitation concept for the mentally retarded. In the remainder of this chapter, I shall discuss the *Wyatt* case, in which the right to habilitation was first articulated, and some of the other recent cases in which the rights of the retarded have been explored.

Wyatt v. Stickney

In October 1970, a class action was filed in federal court in Alabama, alleging that the involuntarily confined mental patients at Bryce State Hospital were being denied their constitutional rights in that they were not being afforded adequate treatment. In August 1971, the class was enlarged to include the mentally retarded residents at the Partlow State School and Hospital. After lengthy hearings the court issued a series of orders in which it found habilitation to be inadequate at Partlow, and set minimum constitutional standards for adequate habilitation.

It is significant that this landmark decision regarding mentally retarded citizens developed literally from a footnote to a decision regarding the mentally ill.[28] The concept of a right to treatment for the mentally ill had been gestating during the preceding years, beginning with the decision in *Rouse v. Cameron*.[29] In the *Rouse* case, the Court of Appeals for the District of Columbia Circuit held that a person involuntarily confined in a public mental hospital had a judicially enforceable right to adequate treatment. While the court based this ruling on a District of Columbia statute, it enumerated constitutional provisions—due process, equal protection, the prohibition of cruel and unusual punishment—that could arguably compel the same result.

The *Rouse* decision triggered much debate in legal and psychiatric circles about the concept of judicial review of the adequacy of treatment of the mentally ill.[30] Prior to that time, it was an unchallenged dogma that the mental hospital administrator was in total control of the quality, kind, and quantity of treatment provided. Even though the involuntary confinement of the administrator's patients was the result of court orders, the courts had not assumed responsibility for assuring that the promised treatment, which justified confinement, was in fact delivered. Notably absent from the professional discussion following *Rouse* was any consideration of the implications of the constitutional issues posed by *Rouse* for the mentally retarded. The failure to make this logical extension of the right-to-treatment principle reflects, in large part, the ignorance of and indifference to the problems of mentally retarded citizens that has characterized the legal profession.

The case of *Wyatt v. Stickney* is a landmark in the effort to improve the treatment of the mentally retarded, to define with particularity the scope of their legal rights, and to assure that their rights are implemented. For the first time, a court recognized that the Constitution provides protection to involuntary mentally retarded residents in public institutions. In finding that the mentally retarded person who is involuntarily confined has a constitutional right to habilitation, the court relied heavily on its previous finding that the mentally ill had a right to treatment: "In the context of the right to appropriate care for people civilly confined to public mental institutions, no viable distinction can be made between the mentally ill and the mentally retarded."[31] The court concluded that the mentally retarded person had "an inviolable constitutional right to habilitation."[32]

After concluding that the right to habilitation was being violated, the court called on the state to propose a plan that would assure that the right was respected. Since the state failed to do so, the court held hearings in which expert testimony was presented concerning the specific minimum components of an adequate habilitation program. The preconditions of such a program were defined: a humane physical and psychological environment; an individual habilitation plan for each resident; an adequate staff in numbers and training to provide habilitation.

An effort was made to frame standards which were sufficiently specific and objective to permit effective judicial administration. Abstract statements of principles or norms in terms of "adequacy" would not provide a suitable benchmark by which a court could measure institutional performance. However, balanced against the concern with objectivity and ease of administration was the need to preserve sufficient flexibility so that habilitation professionals would not be precluded from innovative approaches. It was recognized that the standards would be in need of revision from time to time, in light of evolving habilitation techniques and a new awareness of institutional problems. The standards adopted by the court reflected the best expert opinion at the time the standards were developed, but they were not definitive. For example, no standard was adopted to deal specifically with the problem of sterilization of mentally retarded residents. Subsequent experience at the Partlow School indicated that such a standard was clearly needed. Counsel for plaintiffs raised the issue by amici; and a new standard was adopted by the court. Subsequent analysis of hospital and institutional performance will undoubtedly reveal other areas—the issue of overuse of psychoactive medication, and the problem of obtaining consent to therapy from mentally retarded residents and the like—which will require adoption of additional standards and revision of standards initially adopted.

The principal criticism of the standards adopted by the court is their "lack of realism." Critics note that the standards call for staffing of the institutions with more professionals than there are in the State of Alabama. But, recruitment efforts have by no means been exhausted, and imaginative recruiting might succeed in obtaining much more adequate staffing than had previously been anticipated. More importantly, if the state cannot recruit sufficient staff to provide adequate habilitation services, it should not confine retarded people in institutions for purposes of habilitation. If a state cannot provide habilitation services in a residential setting for thousands of retarded individuals, it should not place so many individuals in the institution. A variety of flexible services to the retarded living in the community would probably be cheaper than full-time institutionalization and it would be more consistent with the proper respect for the constitutional rights of the retarded citizen.

Significantly, the court's standards addressed the need for prompt redress of the horrible conditions in the state institutions for the retarded and also built into its order elements that would lead to reduction of the institutional population and return of its residents to the community. In this respect, the *Wyatt* decision incorporates current thinking among mental retardation professionals regarding habilitation. In adopting the contemporary view that the retarded person should live in conditions that are as close to normal as possible, the court rejected the duality which treated the mentally retarded in the institution as a discrete class, clearly distinguishable from those who were fit to live in the community. The decision incorporates key standards[33] which embody the normalization principle and the notion that the mentally retarded should not, in general, be taken out of the community and placed in massive institutions at all. In Standard 3, for example, the court states:

(a) No person shall be admitted to the institution unless prior determination shall have been made that residence in the institution is the least restrictive habilitation setting feasible for that person. (b) No mentally retarded person shall be admitted to the institution if services and programs in the community can afford adequate habilitation to such persons. (c) Residents shall have a right to the least restrictive conditions necessary to achieve the purposes of habilitation. To this end, the institution shall make every attempt to move residents from (1) more to less structured living; (2) larger to smaller facilities; (3) larger to smaller living quarters; (4) group to individual residence; (5) segregated from the community to integrated into the community; (6) dependent to independent living.[34]

In addition, Standard 4 provides explicitly that no borderline or mildly retarded person shall be a resident at Partlow.[35] Standard 10, stressing that institutionalization is not a final disposition of a hopelessly incompetent person, states that each resident shall have, upon admission, as part of his habilitation plan, an individualized post-institutionalization plan.[36] Standard 47 states that each resident discharged into the community shall have a program of transitional habilitation assistance.[37]

Thus, the court in *Wyatt* addresses the problem of assuring adequate habilitation to institutional residents, at the same time avoiding the pitfall of continuing to accept a dualistic system which necessarily isolates the institution from the community. In addition, while not formally addressing itself to commitment procedures, the order assures that the kinds of people who have been inappropriately placed in the institution in the past will not be institutionalized in the future.

The *Wyatt* decision is now on appeal in the United States Court of Appeals for the Fifth Circuit, and a decision is awaited on the underlying question of the constitutional right to habilitation. Despite the fact that an appeal is still pending, the *Wyatt* decision has had a tremendous impact. Like *Rouse,* it has spawned discussions, symposia, and scholarly debate. It helped loose a series of lawsuits, in numerous states, seeking to vindicate the right to habilitation. It has abetted the ferment within mental health professional organizations. It has made professional and citizen groups concerned with inadequacy of services for the mentally retarded newly conscious of litigation as a method for pursuing their program objectives. It has stimulated state mental health departments to review their own practices and administrative policy in order to stave off litigation. It has helped fuel recent legislative efforts to revise mental health laws.

Other Recent Right-to-Habilitation Cases

Even though the *Wyatt* case is still on appeal, it has been cited as authority in several recent decisions recognizing a constitutional right to habilitation and analogous rights of involuntarily confined people.[38] As the district court stated in *Welsch v. Likins,* after citing the *Wyatt* decision: "There is, in short, a growing body of law recognizing a constitutional right to treatment for persons confined in various settings under State authority without having been found culpable of criminal conduct."[39]

The *Wyatt* approach has not, however, been adopted by all courts faced with the question. In *Burnham v. Department of Public Health,*[40] decided by a federal district court in Georgia in August 1972, plaintiffs alleged inadequate treatment and habilitation in Georgia's mental institutions. The court granted defendants' motion to dismiss, and held that there is no constitutional right to treatment for habilitation. Plaintiffs in that case, inmates of the state's mental institutions, had alleged that they were denied a humane psychological and physical environment, that staff was insufficient to provide adequate treatment, and that there were no individualized treatment plans. The district court refused to hold an evidentiary hearing, emphasizing that the State of Georgia, unlike Alabama, was making large expenditures for its mental health programs. However, the fact that funding levels were generally higher in Georgia than in Alabama could hardly establish that constitutionally acceptable habilitation and treatment programs existed in all the state's institutions.

I have suggested above that the equal protection and due process clauses and the prohibition of cruel and unusual punishment confer substantial protections on the institutionalized mentally retarded. By dismissing plaintiffs' complaint without a hearing, the district court in *Burnham* implied that these constitutional provisions could not be violated upon any kind of factual showing. In the event that the *Burnham* result is sustained on appeal, the development of a right to habilitation by the federal courts could be aborted. (The *Burnham* appeal has been consolidated with the *Wyatt* appeal. Both were argued in December 1972 and await decision.)

One other important case, *New York State Association for Retarded Children v. Rockefeller* (the *"Willowbrook"* case)[41] should be discussed. One year after *Wyatt*, a federal district court in New York entered a preliminary order in this case. The plaintiffs, the state mental retardation association and individual parents, filed suit alleging violations of constitutional rights and seeking a preliminary injunction which would protect the residents of Willowbrook from harm while the decision on the broader issue of adequate habilitation was pending. Hearings were held in December 1972 and in January 1973 on plaintiffs' request for preliminary relief. Unlike the district court in *Burnham*, the judge in *Willowbrook* refused to resolve the legal issues in the abstract, without looking at the facts, stating: "It is very difficult to separate fact from law. And I think it is appropriate that I give the plaintiffs a chance to present their picture so that I can decide the legal issues in light of the actual situation as presented."[42] It is possible that the conditions of gross neglect and deprivation that he found at Willowbrook shaped his decision to order substantial relief. He stated such conditions "are hazardous to the health, safety, and sanity of the residents.[43] Based on this holding, the court entered a wide-ranging decree of April 10, 1973, granting most of the relief plaintiffs had requested. This included a ban on the use of seclusion; a requirement of substantial additions to professional and nonprofessional staff by May 31; and a requirement that appropriate provision for medical attention to acutely ill residents be made. The order went so far as to require that the starting salary for physical therapists be raised in order to permit effective recruitment.

The court noted that its order "may not exhaust the rights to which the federal Constitution entitles residents of a place like Willowbrook."[44] Thus, the court held open the possibility that broader relief would be granted after a full hearing on the merits. Looking to the nature of the relief ordered, the judge's action in *Willowbrook* is analogous to the court's order for emergency relief entered immediately at the end of the *Partlow* hearing.

The conceptual basis for the court's decision to grant preliminary relief in *Willowbrook* is, however, different from the *Wyatt* court's. The decision in *Willowbrook* does not rest on a "right to habilitation." Rather, it finds in the due process, equal protection, and cruel and unusual punishment clauses a right of residents to be protected from harm. The court rejects any distinction between voluntary and involuntary residents for this purpose. The court notes that all the residents are treated alike in the institution,[45] and that they "are for the most part confined behind locked gates; and are held without the possibility of a meaningful waiver of their right to freedom."[46] It further notes that conditions tolerable in prison where punishment is permissible may not be tolerable in institutions for mentally retarded citizens, where punishment is impermissible.[47] The underlying premise behind this analysis appears to be that the retarded residents should be treated as an involuntarily confined population.[48]

This conceptual justification gave the court a sufficient constitutional basis for purposes of the preliminary relief requested by plaintiffs. The court explicitly stated that it did not in its order address all the rights to which the federal Constitution entitles residents of an institution for the mentally retarded.[49] The "protection from harm" standard articulated for the first time in this opinion is extremely open ended. Does it apply to mental as well as physical harm? Is harm to the resident to be measured in terms of actual deterioration, or is it to be measured against the development that a retarded person would have had if he had an adequate habilitation program? Many experts would argue that a resident in a large institution always suffers harm unless an adequate and appropriate habilitation program is developed for him; that without affirmative habilitation efforts a retarded person necessarily regresses in the institution. Most important, many experts would argue that confinement of many retarded persons in institutions like Willowbrook causes harm because of the very nature of the institution, regardless of the adequacy of staffing and programming. Would such confinement then "shock the conscience of the court" or offend "civilized standards of human decency"?[50] It is unclear how the court in *Willowbrook* would respond to these questions.

The preliminary order in *Willowbrook* seems to accept the inherited system of treating the mentally retarded, particularly the notion that habilitation in the institution can be treated in isolation. However, this opinion was based only on plaintiffs' request for preliminary injunction. At a comparable stage in the *Wyatt* proceeding, the court was also concerned with the barbarous conditions in the institutions: the assaults on residents, the acute understaffing, the inadequacy of medical care. When the issue has been presented in full, the nexus between the institution and the community—the necessarily nonhabilitative character of the massive institution, and the inappropriate institutionalization of most residents—may lead the *Willowbrook* court to recognize that the plight of the mentally retarded resident cannot be dealt with simply by improving institutions.

THE RIGHTS OF THE RETARDED AFTER *WYATT*

In appraising the impact of the right-to-habilitation litigation, it is important to see litigation in context, and not to have unrealistic expectations. The *Wyatt* decision illustrates some of the potency and limitations of litigation as a technique. The *Wyatt* order is not self-enforcing. It requires much more than a court order to move a large bureaucracy to solve an intractable problem. No one would assert that all inappropriately placed residents of Partlow have been returned to the community or that adequate habilitation programs have been instituted. But a start has been made, and the orientation of the Department of Mental Health has shifted toward community care.

The response of the Alabama Department of Mental Health in the period following the entry of the order, has reflected an understanding of the need to improve habilitation in the institution while reducing population and developing community alternatives. The Partlow Human Rights Committee, an independent citizen committee established by the court to monitor compliance with the court's order, filed a report on implementation which indicated that the state administrators understood that a primary response to the order must be rapid reduction of the Partlow population. Meeting the minimum physical standards for the institution was explicitly tied to a reduction in population. In the year following the court's order, 500 residents were released, bringing the population down to 1,745. Further reductions to a level of approximately 700 residents were planned. At the same time, the number of qualified mental retardation professionals and the number of resident care workers was doubled, although the level of professional staffing remained woefully inadequate. The Department had begun to develop a range of community services for the mentally retarded, including small group homes.

The Human Rights Committee noted progress in some areas within the institution, but there were still glaring inadequacies, particularly in the fundamental matter of medical care. The Committee urged immediate attention to these inadequacies within the institution but recognized that the long-term resolution of these problems could only come about through reduction in the institutional population and the transformation of the institution's very character.

A judicial order recognizing the right to habilitation and setting out minimum standards is merely the beginning of a long and difficult task. The *Wyatt* decision has acted as a catalyst to mobilize public opinion: effective implementation of the *Wyatt* order will require political action and continuing public attention to the problem.

There are, in addition, discernible secondary consequences which have flowed from judicial intervention in the area of the right to habilitation. It has helped generate a rethinking of the systems that purport to serve mentally retarded individuals and, superimposed on that system, an analysis that stresses the constitutional rights of the mentally retarded citizen. For mental retardation administrators, for parents, and for mentally retarded residents in state institutions, this emphasis on constitutional rights has had substantial consequences.

Mental retardation professionals have had to redefine their roles and professional responsibilities. The administrator of a state institution for the mentally retarded can no longer think he is fulfilling his responsibilities if he runs an adequate custodial program. The fundamental habilitation purposes of such institutions have again been reaffirmed. Many states are now in the process of revising their laws relating to the mentally retarded. The perspectives reflected in recent judicial opinions have helped stimulate and shape such statutory revisions, and have encouraged the development of new legislation. Similarly, new administrative policies being developed within states in many instances are affected by judicial decisions. Several states have used the *Wyatt* standards to measure performance in their own system.

The *Wyatt* decision has also underlined the need to develop community services as an alternative to institutionalization. It has raised the price of institutional warehousing and focused public attention on the inadequacy of institutionalization as a solution. It is likely that the next generation of litigation, building on the right-to-education litigation[51] and the emphasis of the *Wyatt* order on normalization[52] will focus on the quantity and quality of services available to the mentally retarded in the community.[53] In this connection, the most significant consequence of the recent right-to-habilitation litigation may be in raising new questions for exploration rather than in providing the answers.

Adequacy of Community Services

There has been much public debate about the "dumping" of mentally ill and mentally retarded people in the community. In the wake of right-to-habilitation litigation with its emphasis on the transfer of mentally retarded people back to the community, there has been a new focus on this question. Litigation was brought in California, for example, to prohibit the closing of institutions for the mentally retarded before adequate community facilities were established.

In the District of Columbia, suit was filed against the Department of Health, Education, and Welfare and the District of Columbia in order to compel the defendants to establish appropriate community facilities for mentally ill people involuntarily confined in St. Elizabeths Hospital.[54] The defendants themselves had estimated that more than half of the current patients should be placed in alternative, community-based facilities. The suit, which was brought on behalf of several patients and professional organizations, seeks to assure that community facilities will be established and adequately staffed to provide appropriate habilitation programs. Assuring the continuing adequacy of community treatment facilities will be an ongoing problem.

Uncompensated Patient Labor

In the *Wyatt* proceeding, the court ordered an end to involuntary, uncompensated patient labor within the state's mental institution. Subsequently, the suit *Souder v. Brennan*[55] was brought in the District to compel the Department of Labor to enforce minimum wage laws as they applied to mentally ill and mentally retarded persons. The district court held that the minimum wage laws are applicable and that the defendant has an obligation to enforce them. The way in which institutions will adapt to this new situation is yet to be worked out.

Voluntary Admissions

The recent litigation has also raised substantial questions about the way "voluntary" residents of mental institutions should be treated. Since virtually the entire population in the Alabama institutions was involuntary, this was not a critical question in *Wyatt*. However, in many jurisdictions many persons are voluntarily confined. In *Saville v. Treadway*,[56] a three-judge district court held the Tennessee voluntary commitment procedures for the retarded to be unconstitutional. Finding that vital interests of personal liberty were at stake, the court held that adequate procedural protections must be provided before a retarded person is confined in a state institution. The court held further, that the significant potential for conflict of interest between a parent and retarded child precluded the state from presuming that the parent could be reliably expected to adequately represent the child's interests.

The situation of the voluntary resident within the institution has yet to be clarified and resolved. It has been argued that in institutions for the retarded no distinction should be recognized between voluntary and involuntary residents in determining their constitutional rights; there is usually no distinction made between the care afforded to "voluntary" and "involuntary" residents. The two groups are provided the same habilitation services, subjected to the same limitations on movement, and treated with the same impersonality. As the court noted in *Willowbrook*, both "are held without the possibility of a meaningful waiver of their right to freedom."[57] It would be incongruous if constitutional doctrine were interpreted to require that one group was to receive substantially different habilitation services than the other. Initial decisions recognizing rights of mentally retarded citizens in institutions have, in effect, rejected such a distinction.[58]

Sterilization

For many years, sterilization of the mentally retarded was thought to be a suitable technique of improving the genetic stock of the human race. This eugenic theory has since been discredited, but the practice of sterilizing the retarded has not been eliminated. Indeed, more than 20 states still have mandatory sterilization laws on the books.

After the main orders were entered in *Wyatt*, counsel for plaintiffs discovered that sterilizations were still taking place in the Partlow School. Since no standards directly relating to sterilization had previously been adopted, a second round of proceedings was initiated. A three-judge court was convened to consider the Alabama mandatory sterilization law. The court held that the law violated due process in that it failed to establish suitable procedures prior to the sterilization decision. Judge Johnson then issued standards, relying heavily on proposals submitted by the Department of Justice, which assured that sterilizations would not be performed on institutional inmates unless the resident had a "genuine desire" to be sterilized; alternative contraceptive methods had been given full consideration; and the sterilization decision had been reviewed by independent decision makers.

Treatments That Cannot Be Imposed on Mental Patients

The right-to-treatment concept raises questions as to whether residents of mental institutions have a right to be free from certain kinds of treatment. The *Wyatt* decision begins to deal with some kinds of problems of this sort—limiting or prohibiting psychosurgery and other experimental treatments, imposing limitations on behavior modification, particularly with aversive stimuli, and limiting the uses of psychoactive medication. In other lawsuits, these issues are being more fully explored. For example, in *Kaimowitz v. Department of Mental Health*[59] an experimental psychosurgery program in a state mental hospital was challenged. The court held that the conduct of this experimental procedure on an involuntarily confined mental patient violated his constitutional rights. In *Bell v. Wayne County General Hospital at Eloise*,[60] a suit was brought to challenge the use of psychoactive medication on a mental patient, who was held under a temporary detention, prior to adjudication of mental illness. That case is now pending before a three-judge court in Michigan.

In summary, many difficult issues which had not been within the vision of the legal process have been brought into view by the right-to-treatment litigation. We can anticipate that these questions will be dealt with for the next several years, in the courts, in mental health departments, and in state legislatures.

It is impossible to predict the outcome of the litigation involving the right to habilitation of the mentally retarded over the long run. Court orders will not in themselves change the world; civil rights lawyers, welfare reform lawyers, and poverty lawyers have learned this lesson in recent years. But, judicial proceedings can energize concerned communities and mental retardation professionals. These concerned groups must have the will and stamina to seize the opportunity presented by recent judicial attention to the right to habilitation and the other rights of mentally retarded citizens.

NOTES

1. Wyatt v. Stickney, 325 F. Supp. 781 (M. D. Ala. 1971), 334 F. Supp. 1341 (M. D. Ala. 1971), 344 F. Supp. 373, 344 F. Supp. 387 (M. D. Ala. 1972), *appeal docketed sub mon. Wyatt v. Aderholt,* No. 72-2634, 5th Cir. The appeal was argued in December 1972. No decision has been rendered.

2. Habilitation has been defined as "the process by which the staff of the institution assists the resident to acquire and maintain those life skills which enable him to cope more effectively with the demands of his own person and of his environment and to raise the level of his physical, mental, and social efficiency. Habilitation includes but is not limited to programs of formal, structured education and treatment." Wyatt v. Stickney, 344 F. Supp. at 395.

3. See *The Mentally Disabled and the Law* (rev. ed. S. Brakel & R. Rock eds.; Chicago: University of Chicago Press, 1971), pp. 98-102.

4. *Ala. Code* tit. 45, Z 236 (1958).

5. *See, e.g.,* E Goffman, *Asylums* (New York: Doubleday-Anchor, 1961); D. Vail, *Dehumanization and the Institutional Career* (Springfield, Ill.: C. C. Thomas, 1966).

6. Brown v. Board of Education, 347 U.S. 483 (1954).

7. The following discussion draws heavily on the legal analysis in the brief in the court of appeals in the Wyatt case filed by amici curiae, American Association on Mental Deficiency, American Civil Liberties Union, American Orthopsychiatric Association, American Psychological Association, National Association for Mental Health, National Association for Retarded Children, and the American Psychiatric Association.

8. Speiser v. Randahl, 357 U.S. 513, 525 (1958).

9. See Covington v. Harris, 419 F. 2d 617, 623 (D. C. Cir. 1969); Lessard v. Schmidt, 349 F. Supp. 1078 (E. D. Wisc. 1972), *vacated and remanded,* 42 U.S.L.W. 3402 (U.S. Jan. 14, 1974) (The Supreme Court made no ruling on the merits, but rather vacated the

order below as being insufficiently specific in the formulation of its remedy); *cf.* Wolf v. Colorado, 338 U.S. 25, 27 (1949).

10. *See, e.g.,* Goffman, *op. cit.;* Vail, *op. cit.*

11. This discussion refers to *involuntarily* confined retarded persons. The argument for treating all mentally retarded persons in institutions as involuntary residents is set out below.

12. Jackson v. Indiana, 406 U.S. 715 (1972).

13. 406 U.S. at 738. *See also* McNeil v. Director, Patuxent Institution, 407 U.S. 245 (1072).

14. 325 F. Supp. at 784.

15. The fact that some mentally retarded persons may be thought to be dangerous to society does not relieve the state of its obligation to assure adequate habilitation if they are committed to institutions for the retarded. *See* Tippett v. Maryland, 436 F. 2d 1153 (4th Cir. 1971); Kent v. United States, 401 F. 2d 408, 411-12 (D. C. Cir. 1968); Inmates of the Boys Training School v. Affleck, 346 F. Supp. 1354 (D. R. I. 1972); Commonwealth v. Page, 339 Mass. 313, 159 N. E. 2d 82 (1959).

16. Hamilton v. Love, 328 F. Supp. 1182, 1193 (E. D. Ark. 1971).

17. Rozecki v. Gaughan, 459 F.2d 6 (1st Cir. 1972). *See also* Cross v. Harris, 418 F.2d 1095, 1101 (D. C. Cir. 1969) ("Incarceration may not seem 'punishment' to the jailors but it is punishment to the jailed."); United States *ex rel.* Schuster v. Herold, 410 F.2d 1071, 1090-91 (2d Cir. 1969) (detailed comparison showing conditions in Massachusetts mental institution more restrictive than prison); Inmates of Boys Training School v. Affleck, 346 F. Supp. 1354 (D. R. I. 1972); United States *ex rel.* von Wolfersdorf v. Johnson, 317 F. Supp. 66 (S. D. N. Y. 1970).

18. Robinson v. California, 370 U.S. 660 (1962); Trop v. Dulles, 356 U.S. 86, 101 (1958) ("There may be involved no physical mistreatment . . . . There is instead the total destruction of the individual's status in organized society.").

19. Robinson v. California, 370 U.S. 660, 666 (1962). The Supreme Court has cautioned against evasion of the eighth amendment standard by the adoption of sham treatment programs—"the hanging of a new sign reading 'hospital' over one wing of the jailhouse." Powell v. Texas, 392 U.S. 514, 529 (1968). *See also* Easter v. District of Columbia, 361 F.2d 50, 55 (D. C. Cir. 1966); Driver v. Hinnant, 356 F.2d 761, 765 (4th Cir. 1966) (Incarceration of chronic alcoholics for status constitutes cruel and unusual punishment but detention for treatment and rehabilitation is permissible).

20. 334 F. Supp. at 1343; 344 F. Supp. at 393-394.

21. *See* Haines v. Kerner, 404 U.S. 519 (1972); Wright v. McMann, 387 F.2d 519 (2d Cir. 1967); Jones v. Wittenberg, 323 F. Supp. 93 (N. D. Ohio 1971); Hancock v. Avery, 301 F. Supp. 786 (M. D. Tenn. 1969).

22. *See* Dunn v. Blumstein, 405 U.S. 330 (1972). *See also* "Developments in the Law—Equal Protection," *Harv. L. Rev.,* 82 (1969), 1065.

23. *Cf.* Speiser v. Randall, 357 U.S. 513, 525 (1958). *See also* Williams v. Illinois, 399 U.S. 235, 263 (1970) (Harlan, J., concurring); Chambers, "Alternatives to Civil Commitment of the Mentally Ill—Practical Guides and Constitutional Imperatives," *Mich. L. Rev.,* 70, (1972), 1107, 1155-68.

24. The Supreme Court has placed great emphasis on the right to travel. Papachristou v. City of Jacksonville, 405 U.S.156, 163-64 (1972); Aptheker v. Secretary of State, 378 U.S.500 (1964); Kent v. Dulles, 357 U.S. 116, 125 (1958).Similarly, the court has protected the right to free association. Coates v. City of Cincinnati, 402 U.S. 611 (1971).

25. *See, e.g., Ala. Code* tit. 45, ZZ 231-52 (a16) (Supp. 1971).

26. Baxtrom v. Herold, 383 U.S. 107, 111 (1966).

27. *Id.* at 115.

28. Wyatt v. Stickney, 334 F. Supp. 1341, n. 1.

29. Rouse v. Cameron, 373 F. 2d 451 (D. C. Cir. 1966).

30. E. G., Tribby v. Cameron, 379 F.2d 104 (D. C. Cir. 1967); Nason v. Superintendent of Bridgewater State Hosp., 353 Mass. 604, 223 N. E. 2d 908 (1968); D. Bazelon, "Implementing the Right to Treatment," *U. Chi. L. Rev.*, 36 (1969), 742; "Symposium: The Right to Treatment," Geo. L. J., 57 (1969) 673; Note, "The Nascent Right to Treatment," *Va. L. Rev.*, 53 (1967), 1134; Note, "Civil Restraint, Mental Illness, and the Right to Treatment," *Yale L. J.* 77 (1967), 87; Council of the American Psychiatric Association, "Position Paper on the Question of Adequacy of Treatment," *Amer. J. Psychiatry, 123 (1967), 1458.*

31. 344 F. Supp. at 390.

32. Id.

33. The court's standards are set out at 344 F. Supp. at 395-407.

34. 344 F. Supp. at 396.

35. Id.

36. Id. at 397.

37. Id. at 407.

38. Welsch v. Likins, No. 4-72-Civ. 451 (D. Minn.), dec. Feb. 15, 1974 (mentally retarded have constitutional right to habilitation); Morales v. Turman, Civ. No. 1948 (E. D. Tex.) interim order issued Aug. 31, 1973 (juveniles); Stachulak v. Coughlin, 364 F. Supp. 686 (N. D. Ill. 1973) (sexually dangerous persons); Nelson v. Heyne, Civ. Nos. 72-1970, 73-1446 (7th Cir.) dec. Jan. 31, 1974 (juveniles).

39. Welsch v. Likins, No. 4-72-Civ. 451 (D. Minn.), slip op. p. 11.

40. Burnham v. Department of Public Health, 349 F. Supp. 1335 (M. D. Ga. 1972).

41. New York State Association for Retarded Children v. Rockefeller, 357 F. Supp. 752 (E. D. N. Y. 1973).

42. Transcript, Hearing on Preliminary Injunction, at 7.

43. 357 F. Supp. at 765.

44. Id.

45. 357 F. Supp. at 756.

46. 357 F. Supp. at 764.

47. Id.

48. Noting that there may be a conflict between the interest of a parent in committing a retarded child and the best interests of the child, the court states "A 'voluntary admission' on the petition of parents may quite properly be treated in the same category as an 'involuntary admission' in the absence of evidence that the child's interests have been fully considered." 357 F. Supp. at 762.

49. 357 F. Supp. at 765.

50. Id.

51. Mills v. Board of Education, 348 F. Supp. 866 (1972).

52. 344 F. Supp. at 399-405.

53. *See* Robinson v. Weinberger, Civ. No. 285-74, filed February 14, 1974 (D. D. C.) (complaint alleging that patients improperly confined in mental hospitals have institutional and statutory right to placement in suitable community-based facility).

54. Id.

55. Souder v. Brennan, C.A. No. 482-72 (D.D.C.), Dec. Nov. 14, 1973.

56. Saville v. Treadway, Civ. Action No. 6969 (M. D. Tenn.), dec. Mar. 8, 1974.

57. 357 F. Supp. at 764.

58. This type of inequity was avoided by the United States District Court for the District of Massachusetts (Ford, J.) when it denied (without opinion) the state's motion to dismiss for lack of jurisdiction. The court rejected the state's contention that the quality of service provided by the state to voluntary residents of the Belchertown State School was not of constitutional dimensions and therefore not properly before the court. Ricci v. Greenblatt, Civil No. 72-469-F (D. Mass., Mar. 13, 1972). In Wyatt, the court stated that

its holding applied only to involuntary residents. (There were, as a practical matter, only a few residents at Partlow who had been admitted to the institution by the procedure denominated "voluntary.") The court, however, presumed that the right to habilitation applied to *all* residents, and stated that the institution had the "difficult burden" of proving that any particular resident had not been involuntarily committed. 344 F. Supp. at 390 n.5. By this analysis, the court implied that the right to habilitation is applicable to all residents, absent a showing of genuine voluntariness.

In the Willowbrook case, the court held that all residents of Willowbrook should receive the same protection without regard to the statutory procedure by which they were admitted.

59. *Prison Law Reporter,* 2 (July 1973).

60. Bell v. Wayne County General Hospital at Eloise, C. A. No. 36384 (E. D. Mich.).

The Core Problem Controversy

STUART GOLANN

One recurring issue of mental health social policy is the "core problem controversy."[1] Specifically, should priority be given to those persons now significantly impaired or should more resources be devoted to the prevention of impairment? Every time a new social policy initiative occurs in the mental health field, this controversy reappears in one or more ways. The following chapter by Stuart Golann asks what effect the reconstruction of mental health service standards through constitutional law will have on priorities within the mental health fields.

Dr. Golann considers the sources of the core problem controversy and cautions against the inadvertent use of constitutional law to strengthen an effective custodial model of patient care. He concludes the chapter by asking the reader to consider two questions which underlie the paradox of right-to-treatment reform.

Nowhere has the inadequacy of mental hospital treatment been more directly addressed than in the 1961 final report of the Joint Commission on Mental Illness and Health. The Commission had been directed by Congress to analyze and evaluate the needs and resources of the mentally ill in the United States and make recommendations for a national mental health program. They concluded that:

If we are to be wholly honest with ourselves and with the public, then we must view the mental health problem in terms of the unmet need—those who are untreated and inadequately cared for. We have no definitive analysis of how many such patients there are, but information we have leads us to believe that more than half of the patients in most State hospitals receive no active treatment of any kind designed to improve their mental condition.[2]

Consequently, the Joint Commission recommended that a national mental health program should recognize major mental illness as the core problem and that intensive treatment of patients with critical and prolonged mental breakdowns should have first call on fully trained members of the mental health professions. The Commission also stated that the "risk of false promise" would be avoided if public education for better mental health focused on disseminating information about mental illness which the public needs and wants in order to recognize psychological forms of sickness and arrive at an informed opinion of its responsibility toward the mentally ill.[3]

One of a number of criticisms of the Joint Commission's report appeared in the newsletter *Alabama Mental Health* in an article titled "The Risk of False Promise in Achieving Public Emotional Well-Being."[4] In this article, T. H. Stubbs rejected an either-treatment-or-prevention formulation of national mental health policy, criticizing as particularly regrettable the setting up of a dichotomy that divided mental health functions into treatment and mental health education. He said further, that it discredits education to confuse it with the passing on of information from those who know to those who don't know; instead of such a limited formulation of mental health education, he suggested that the reinforcement of the entire range of community resources is as important a task for professional manpower as the treatment of the sick. No disease, he held, has ever been conquered simply by treating individuals who were sick with it. Instead, he advocated searching for more adequate methods of providing life experiences which decrease disturbed human relationships and assure the optimal level of health for the total population.

The "core problem controversy" between proponents of prevention and advocates of treatment preceded the Joint Commission report and has continued ever since. The same basic controversy may be seen in the early history of the mental hygiene movement, in the formation of policy for child guidance centers, mental hospitals, and the more recent community mental health centers. This chapter explores why there has been a core problem controversy and how possible judicial intervention into the mental health system may affect it.

SOURCES OF THE CORE PROBLEM CONTROVERSY

At one important level, the core problem controversy is a battle over social and professional helping priorities. At another level it may be viewed as the operational expression of a basic ideologic rift between biological and social psychological concepts of behavior disorder. Feeding the controversy at both levels are problems of vested interests and power conflicts; limited goal definitions and inadequate consideration of strategy alternatives for achieving mental health program goals; and inadequate resources—especially manpower and technology—requiring, in the absence of clear goals and results, that priorities be established politically.

Ideologic Dissonance in Mental Health

In the historic evolution of mental health ideology, supernatural and demonic explanations of personal torment or unusual behavior gave way to moral-humanistic and next to scientific-physiological orientations. These in turn were supplemented or replaced by psychodynamic and interpersonal concepts. Today, mental health specialists increasingly seek explanations for individual behavior in the political and social institutions which mediate individual development, adaptation, and satisfaction. The community resources that are called upon to influence behavior at any time in history are determined by the assumptions of the prevailing ideologic position—especially the key assumption of what lies behind or causes the problem behavior. Mechanic, too, has pointed out in a preceding chapter the major ideologies which have shaped the development of mental health services in the United States.

Moral treatment as a form of mental health ideology left a rich and, until recently, overlooked heritage; but successful application of its techniques appears to have been linked to a sympathetic relationship between the help producers and small numbers of service recipients. The scientific-physiological approach to disordered behavior also has a history of partial success—notably that associated with general paresis. While some problems yielded to a biological approach, many more problems have not responded to a biological or medical treatment; the unavailability of alternatives has forced many persons in states of crisis to choose between hospitalization or no services.

Dynamic psychology and psychoanalysis resulted in the application of mental health ideology to a much broadened scope of human behavior, but the applicability of its intervention techniques has not satisfied either the increased demand for services or expectations for equitable service availability.

Social psychological concepts of behavior disorder, the need for more equitable and effective means of providing helping services, and the necessity to balance patient care and prevention of disorder have resulted in what has been alternatively called community psychology and psychiatry, community mental health, or public health-mental health; focus has shifted from the intrapsychic, to the interpersonal, to the broader social networks that are presumed to shape behavior. Classification approaches are shifting from symptomatic classification or classification of intrapersonal psychodynamics to concern for social adaptation and the place of the person in a social system. Existing definitions of mental health and illness are being questioned and may give way to more unitary concepts of competence[5] or of learning how to cope[6] or of the importance of support systems in maintaining socially valued behavior.[7]

Dissonance between community oriented approaches and earlier ideologic positions is apparent in the goals, manpower, services, target populations, timing of services and geographic placement of service programs. The basic paradigm or ideology determines each of these and shapes the whole into a congruent system. Just as the prayers and rituals of the shaman were exposed in an appropriate idiom and strategically congruent with the belief that the disturbed person was possessed, so the differential diagnosis and chemical treatment of the physician in a mental hospital were conceptualized within the idiom of medical science and consistent with the belief that the person suffered from biologic illness. The goal of the shaman was to beat the devil out of the person—the goal of the physician was to cure the disease bringing about change in its natural history.

The goal of a community or public health approach is to work within community systems so that they function to develop and sustain the competence and satisfaction of the individuals who are part of them. Prevention of hospitalization and minimization of the length and totality of any removal from one's normal milieu are related goals. Just as it would have been incongruent to use the strategies of the shaman to achieve the goals of medical science in a mental hospital, so it would be incongruent to use the strategies of the disease model of medical science to achieve the goals of effectiveness in the modern community.

Hobbs[8] has spoken of the recent movement into the community as mental health's third revolution. History may see it as such, but we experience it as a gradual evolution—sometimes frustratingly slow. The institutions toward which reform is directed shape and may preempt resulting change; this theme runs through all the chapters of this book, sometimes as paradox. Fremouw's point that the *Wyatt* standards, if enforced, would strengthen a medical-custodial treatment approach is expanded by Mechanic's quiet observation that right to treatment endorses medical as opposed to other explanations of the conflict between individual and community. The *Wyatt* standards, in Stickney's analysis, may be a backward step in catering to professional prestige rather than effective services; and Halpern states that the effort to assure habilitation in massive institutions for the retarded should not deflect attention from the fact that those institutions themselves are an anachronism.

Why do we hesitate to endorse a medical explanation of deviance or add to the legitimacy of institutions for the mentally ill or retarded? Why are we all drawn so surely into the perplexing ideologic controversies of the mental health field?

Each of us—lawyer, physician, psychologist, sociologist—must answer this question for himself. For myself, the answer is that current ideology and vested interests have limited new ideas and experimentation with new helping strategies and that this is intolerable. Typically, we think of innovation as influencing only treatment choice; but treatment of choice is only one dimension of mental health service strategy. In fact, reluctance to innovate includes an unwillingness to experiment with new sources of manpower (such as clergymen and college students); with populations known to need services but who don't ordinarily seek them (such as the poor and uneducated or people in crisis states); with service locations (such as elementary schools or shopping centers); and with the timing or occasions of service delivery (such as following the loss of a spouse).

The lack of experimentation might be slightly less discouraging if there were reason to belive that mental hospitals adequately help seriously disordered persons. But there is evidence to suggest that they do not help, and there is reason to belive that many persons are harmed by the hospital experience. We have direct observation of what takes place inside the hospital—impressions of no active treatment such as those reported by the Joint Commission; case studies brought to light by lawyers and others investigating the treatment afforded committed persons; and sociological and social psychological study of institution structure, function and interaction patterns within the hospital such as that of Belknap,[9] Goffman,[10] and more recently Braginsky et al.[11] and Rosenhan.[12]

How are we to interpret Rosenhan's finding that when approached by a pseudopatient who asked a question about privileges or staffing, 71 percent of the psychiatrists and 88 percent of the nurses in psychiatric hospitals did not stop to answer the question or look at the person who asked it? Each of these lines of investigation is consistent in suggesting that the hospital is not therapeutic for most patients, and is harmful to many in terms of enforced dependence, powerlessness, and depersonalization.

That our helping strategies in general are insufficient emerged clearly from the Midtown Manhattan studies.[13] Of those adults living at home judged to be "partially or totally incapacitated" (defined as having serious emotional symptom formation and functioning with great difficulty, or being seriously incapacitated, unable to function), only 35 percent had ever been patients in any private or public mental health service. The fact is that the majority of seriously emotionally handicapped persons in this country have never been seen by any of the mental health agencies.

If we allow these lines of evidence to converge, we see that most persons with disabling emotional problems are not reached by public or private mental health services and that our major service institution, the psychiatric hospital, probably harms more than it helps.

If one shortcoming is common to the major orientations that have shaped the mental health field in America, it has been an overcommitment to the validity of one set of explanatory concepts and methods of intervention coupled with intolerance and suspicion of competing points of view. As each school of thought dominated the field, the result had invariably been an insufficient and artificially limited range of helping alternatives traceable, in part, to limited public support coupled with exclusive professional concern with one approach to helping. Unnecessary limitations have been imposed on types of helpers or types of clients, or there has been adherence to fixed preconditions in the location or timing of helping services. The diversity of categories of classification, theories of causation, and techniques of intervention which have been brought forth in past centuries is such as to give pause to the advocate of any particular system. The answer to mental health problems, obviously, does not lie with any one approach. Yet, ideologies are held or abandoned at times when it would appear that alternative courses should have been followed.

The tenacity with which ideologies are held to despite apparent lack of validity and the relative ease with which successful programs of moral treatment gave way to custodial hospitalization may present a paradox unless one recognizes that in all periods of history mental health programming has been influenced by intolerance of differences among people or the politics of wealth and power. Mental health services have at times been rigid and inflexible because preferred service strategies maintained positions of privilege for the helpers instead of being planned for those who needed help.

In the past, conflict over power in mental health institutions or in the determination of national mental health policy has been primarily between different professional groups or groups of different orientation within a limited number of professions. Today the conflict has broadened to include community control as opposed to professional control over service-giving institutions.

THE EFFECTS OF RIGHT-TO-TREATMENT LAWSUITS

The effects of the federal judiciary's intervention in this power conflict are uncertain. None of the professions or representatives of the community are sufficiently committed to evaluation of mental health programs, and Stickney's call for a court-supervised program evaluation effort is unlikely to materialize. In the past, the determinants of program survival or abandonment have almost always been particularistic.

In terms of the core controversy the general problem is that there is no formula to determine what proportion of national resources should be devoted to mental health programs and what proportion of those resources devoted to mental health should be allotted to prevention as opposed to the treatment of already identified cases of disorder. Such allocation is not possible because defined and generally accepted goals do not exist and the validity of both preventive and treatment oriented approaches is not determined sufficiently to establish priorities based upon comparative outcomes.

In addition, resources are limited. In *Wyatt,* when the costs for manpower and facilities are approximated, they appear to be so large that one must ask how state legislatures and taxpayers will respond.

The immediate responses of some states have been to accelerate the placement of patients into community residences, nursing homes, halfway houses, etc. As states are faced with meeting standards of institutional care, thousands of patients may be pushed out of inadequate institutions into the community. Judicial intervention in institutions may not guarantee costly adequate treatment for most patients, but cause scattering of people to myriads of equally inadequate but less expensive and less observable alternatives. Halpern's prediction that the next generation of litigation will focus on community services points up both the inefficiency and the necessity of legal reform.

CONCLUSION: PROBLEMS THAT MUST BE CONSIDERED

First, there is the problem of the discrepancy between existing human service resources and the projected costs of *Wyatt*-type standards. Second, given adequate resources, how to transform these into adequate treatment? And who shall define what is "adequate" and what is "treatment"? Third, how can community mental health services be made adequate given the catalytic and probably simultaneously undermining effect of right-to-treatment litigation on community-based mental health services? Specifically, accelerated hospital discharge rates and reduced admissions will increase the need for community services while standards for adequate institutions will make it more difficult to obtain funds for community services, and especially difficult for preventive services.

Finally, we may ask two questions that appear to underlie the paradox of right-to-treatment reform. One: Are institutionalized persons sick, and if they are not what is the appropriate treatment? Related to this is the second question: For what sickness is the current mode of institutional treatment appropriate?

NOTES

1. In 1961 the Joint Commission on Mental Illness and Health recommended that "A national mental health program should recognize that major mental illness is the core problem and unfinished business of the mental health movement. . . . "

2. Joint Commission on Mental Illness and Health, *Action for Mental Health* (New York: Basic Books, 1961), pp. 22-23.

3. *Ibid.*, p. xvii.

4. T. H. Stubbs, "The Risk of False Promise in Achieving Public Emotional Well-being," *Alabama Mental Health* (Feb.-Mar. 1963), pp. 3-6.

5. K. Menninger, *The Vital Balance* (New York: Viking, 1964) and R. W. White, "Motivation Reconsidered: The Concept of Competence," *Psychological Review,* 66 (1959), 297-333.

6. A. Bandura, "Behavioral Psychopathology," *Scientific American,* 216 (1967), 86ff.

7. G. Caplan, *Support Systems and Community Mental Health* (New York: Behavioral Publications, 1973).

8. N. Hobbs, "Mental Health's Third Revolution," *American Journal of Ortho-psychiatry, 34 (1964),* 1-20.

9. I. Belknap, *Human Problems of a State Mental Hospital* (New York: McGraw-Hill, 1956).

10. E. Goffman, *Asylums, Essays on the Social Situations of Mental Patients and Other Inmates* (Garden City, N.Y.: Doubleday-Anchor, 1961).

11. B. Braginsky, D. Braginsky and K. Ring, *Methods of Madness* (New York: Holt, 1969).

12. D. L. Rosenhan, "On Being Sane in Insane Places," *Science,* 179 (1973), 250-57.

13. L. Srole, T. S. Langer, S. T. Michael, M. K. Opler and T. A. Rennie, *Mental Health in the Metropolis* (New York: McGraw-Hill, 1962).

Perspectives on the Right to Treatment

WILLIAM J. FREMOUW

The concluding chapter summarizes the major points raised at the conference. The first section of the chapter reviews the general legal issues of right to treatment discussed by the judges and lawyers at the conference. The second section traces the deliberation of several groups over the problems of defining standards for treatment. The next section reports participants' broader perspectives of the long-term effects of right-to-treatment litigation. Concepts of treatment and interventions reflecting the major tenets of community mental health are discussed in the legal context of a right to treatment. In the final section, the general consensus of the conference, that long-term changes require a broad, multidimensional attack, is discussed. From this call for new strategies, new coalitions, and new responsibilities for the various participants of the mental health system, more specific suggestions emerged for changing the mental health system.

THE LEGAL AND SOCIAL ISSUES OF THE RIGHT TO TREATMENT

We're dealing with people in a place, not patients in hospitals—we're dealing in social problems, not simply society's response to mental illness.

BENJAMIN BRAGINSKY

The case of *Wyatt v. Stickney* first established a constitutional right to treatment based on the *quid pro quo* interpretation of the basis of involuntary commitment. The historical and legal development of the concept is described by Fremouw in detail in Chapter 1. Judge Johnson ruled that the deprivation of a person's liberty through civil commitment procedures without full legal protection, necessitates that the person receive something in exchange for the loss of freedom. In this context, minimum standards for staff, physical facilities and individualized treatment are required in exchange for the loss of liberty that accompanies involuntary confinement. Judge Johnson's standards became the first judicial definition of mental hospital treatment. However, several months later, an interim emergency order in the *Willowbrook* case created a second and more limited interpretation of the right to treatment. In *Wyatt v. Stickney,* Judge Johnson had affirmed the right of an involuntarily committed person to reside in an adequately staffed and supplied facility, and to receive minimum types of individualized treatment designed for his benefit. The Willowbrook order of Judge Judd recognized only an individual's right to be protected from harm; both the protection of society from dangerous people and the care and treatment of impaired individuals are cited as the constitutional bases for commitment. However, several conference participants maintained that the social control function of commitment, regardless of considerations for the individual, is inescapable.

The question of the legal basis for involuntary commitment led to considering a "right to treatment" as a question of a "right to confine." *Who* has the power to confine *whom where* for *what* purpose, emerged as an underlying legal and social question of the right to treatment. Some predicted that a potential effect of a judicially-defined right to treatment may be to make more explicit the social control function of involuntary commitment, thus ending the disguised use of mental hospitals to control deviance under the guise of treatment for mental illness.

Related to this, it was suggested that a right to treatment could limit the breadth of the mental health system. Economic and legal contingencies would make alternative social control systems less expensive. In the future, individuals may be directed into penal institutions for social control purposes if judicial intervention makes mental institutions too expensive. In short, the right to treatment may begin to close the ever-widening doors into the mental health system.

In these discussions, people debated the fundamental questions surrounding the validity and utility of a medical-intrapsychic model of mental illness to effectively treat an unskilled, uneducated population which becomes institutionalized. "Mental illness" was defined by some participants as the behavior the community labels unacceptable of people unable to cope and function in certain contexts. In their view, this change in the ideology of mental illness necessitates different concepts, different goals, different assessments and different measures of outcome than dictated by the medical model. In spite of acknowledged misuse of the traditional medical model, a few participants warned of the premature rejection of this model of mental illness in favor of a "social deviance" concept.

As basic concepts of mental illness were debated, several participants strongly asserted the need to clearly distinguish mental retardation from mental illness. Paralleling those rejecting the medical model of mental illness, those participants working in mental retardation advocated the development of new concepts, goals and treatments for the mentally retarded different from those previously generated by the medical model. From several perspectives, participants stated that until specific operational goals are defined for each human service system, individuals will continue to be arbitrarily labeled and placed in interchangeable "containers" such as jails, mental hospitals or schools for the retarded. Can those goals be specified? Ultimately, the long-range effect of the right to treatment depends upon the further development and examination of the underlying concepts of mental illness and mental retardation.

STANDARDS FOR ADEQUATE TREATMENT

Demonstrate the effectiveness and sincerity of your benevolence—otherwise don't use it . . .

FEDERAL JUDGE MORRIS LASKER

Benevolence of society toward the mentally ill and retarded is often cited as one basis for involuntary commitment. Beginning with the *Wyatt* class action suit, courts are faced with the problem of defining standards of adequate treatment for thousands of involuntarily committed people. Unlike previous individual cases such as *Rouse* or *Nason*, adequate treatment rather than release from institution is the plaintiff's legal prayer. After 3 days of expert testimony from the major mental health professional organizations, Judge Johnson ordered minimum standards for staffing, physical facilities and individualized treatment plans as necessary for adequate treatment. These standards became the focus of extended discussion during the conference. They were generally criticized as neither necessary nor sufficient for adequate treatment. In general, these standards order an extensive, medically-oriented model of treatment without any guarantee as to the results of inputting these human and physical resources. The majority of participants agreed that too little is known of the relationship between the input of mental health resources and the output of effective treatment to justify ordering just delineated input standards. Instead, some argued (see Stickney, Chapter 2) that standards should establish the *output* of the mental health system and allow the states to use their resources in creative, innovative combinations instead of supplementing a specific institutional model. In an era of slowly emerging community alternatives to institutions, the mandating of minimum resources to institutions was viewed as threatening the forces of progress away from institutional care. In response, several participants in the *Wyatt* case pointed out that the standards permitted flexibility and use of resources or deployment, the only limit being the necessity to petition the court for permission.

In the general discussion of the merits of input versus output standards, one point in particular was emphasized. No semblance of adequate treatment as measured by outcome standards can exist if the institution does not provide the minimum resources for humane care of its residents. Logically, some minimum input of resources, perhaps to meet standards of protection from harm, were considered necessary before any standards of effectiveness could be obtained. Some consensus emerged that standards should include both minimum input as well as output or effectiveness criteria. However, the input standards of necessary resources for humane care must be legally and conceptually separated from the output standards of effective treatment. Otherwise, some warned, standards of both minimum humane care and effective treatment may be abandoned if the treatment does not meet effectiveness criteria. To create adequate treatment, standards of minimum care must be developed and retained while programs for treatment and standards for treatment effectiveness evolve from contemporary models of mental health.

The use of effectiveness standards raises several practical problems. First, to assess effectiveness of an institution or mental health system the goals of the system must be operationally defined. With involuntary commitment, the goal of protection of society from dangerous people as well as the treatment of the individual have been intertwined. To establish output criteria for the mental health system, states would be forced to face conflicts between goals for individual treatment and goals for social regulation of behavior. The complex questions of the cost benefits of treatment to the individual as well as to society in terms of productivity or cost of deviance would emerge.

The definition of program goals for outcome measures of effectiveness also forced consideration of basic ideological questions about mental illness. Alternative explanations of mental illness such as possession by the devil, intrapsychic conflict, biochemical disorder, inadequate learning, social incompetence or sociopolitical labeling obviously yield diverse goals for treatment. Discussion implied that before output standards for an adequate treatment could be developed, many complex ideological issues must be addressed by both suppliers and consumers of the mental health system. The questions created by right to treatment again remain unresolved until more fundamental issues are considered.

If these ideological problems could be resolved, the development of effectiveness criteria would allow cost analyses of mental health programs. Enthusiasm emerged as cost effectiveness and cost benefit data for programs were seen to stimulate accountability of the mental health system to judges, legislators and society. Mental health evaluation has previously been argued according to the *social* benefit to society. Now, *cost* benefit arguments are viewed as necessary to entice cautious legislators into new investments in the mental health system. However, although costs are easy to define, the problem and complexity remains the definition and assessment of personal-social benefits of treatment. Thus in this discussion, the fundamental ideological issues again emerged as inextricably linked to the right to treatment.

Many people acknowledged that the absence of effectiveness data has left the mental health profession without much political leverage to stimulate added investments by state legislators. If program goals could be defined, careful cost benefit analyses of institutional and community programs would allow informed decisions as to treatment models and settings. In this view, cost benefit data would probably increase the use of alternatives to institutionalization instead of buttressing already archaic institutional care.

Amidst the complexities of issues and questions at the conference, one thing emerged clearly. At this point no one knows enough about the long-range effectiveness of most mental health programs, especially community programs, to determine the directions public mental health policy should take. However, complexity in evaluation should not be used as an excuse to avoid this overdue evaluation and accounting of the mental health system. The legal profession involved in the right to treatment requested, implored, and at times demanded the development of this information to insure an intelligent approach to right to treatment.

A BROADER VIEW OF A RIGHT TO TREATMENT

Justice may require immediate, massive remediation, but reason may require immediate, massive organization.

GOTTLIEB SIMON

To several participants, the right to treatment is ultimately considered as one aspect of a broader right to receive adequate health care. Does each American have a right to medical care, treatment and resources to maximize his health and life? Broad social legislation such as Medicare and Medicaid and the recent addition of kidney machine treatment to Social Security reflects social aspirations of widely increased health services.

Can a right to treatment be extended so far as to imply a right to voluntary care? Will anyone in the community with a mild phobia, marital discord or a retarded child have a right to demand mental health services? Some wondered if, in an era of a right to health, mental hospitals will become resorts or retreats for those who request a rest from stressful experiences or boring jobs. These intriguing questions were considered as issues of general social policy and priorities. The ability of the courts to extend the concept of right to treatment on constitutional grounds was viewed as limited to issues surrounding involuntary commitment. Legal experts stated that further authority to enlarge the right to treatment must be derived from legislation defining a statutory right to treatment or health. Therefore, they said, a more general right to treatment and right to health will remain a broader social, legislative policy that must be attacked with strategies other than litigation.

In addition to a right to health, other general issues emerged during the group discussions. As states are faced with meeting standards of institutional care, thousands of patients may be pushed out of inadequate institutions into the community. Judicial intervention in institutions may not guarantee costly adequate treatment for most patients but cause the scattering of these people to myriads of equally inadequate, but less expensive and less observable, alternatives. The assumption that institutions are bad and community alternatives are good was debated and amended by the concept of a good institution and bad community (see Mechanic, Chapter 3, and Golann, Chapter 5). Current right-to-treatment litigation is focusing resources at one point of the mental health system. Many participants warned that the concentration of limited resources at one point in a system will inevitably create shortages in other areas.

The broader question became how an effective, responsive mental health system can be developed. Several participants proposed that instead of razing institutions, institutions should be transformed into humane, constructive facilities that supply necessary services at one point on a continuum of services. To achieve this goal, the development of new models and concepts of institutions are necessary. The discussants agreed that the arbitrary dichotomy between institutions and community alternatives should be replaced by a comprehensive continuum of mental health services from institutional care to minimal community support services as first recommended by the Joint Commission on Mental Illness and Health in 1961.

The concept of treatment in the "least restrictive alternative" established in *Wyatt* was considered as beginning to broaden the judicial intervention into community placement. According to this idea, the treatment any individual receives must be minimally restrictive of his freedom. For example, no one found incompetent to stand trial should be institutionalized if halfway house care would be sufficient to meet treatment goals.

The expansion of a right to treatment from institution to community facilities requires the enormous task of developing new input and effectiveness standards for community care, new models of treatment and new resources. Again, underlying concepts of mental illness and health have to be considered first. For the concept of community treatment to become viable, several people said that community alternatives require a superstructure of support services and resources that do not currently exist. Just as institutions were once heralded as effective, benevolent places for treatment of mental illness during the era of moral therapy, the community is now declared the best setting for adequate treatment. Paradoxically, unless community resources change and grow as concepts of treatment evolve, the community alternatives of halfway houses, welfare hotels and rest homes may become the mini-institutions of dehumanizing care while institutions begin to provide adequate treatment to the few remaining patients. Most participants agreed that the negative cycle can be prevented only by intervention at all points along the mental health system.

The last century of efforts has been devoted to treatment of individuals already severely incapacitated. Instead of tertiary treatment, several participants shared Golann's view in Chapter 5, that secondary or short-term intervention, and especially primary prevention, should be supported to prevent perpetuating a system of costly ineffective intervention. From their perspective, a system of prevention of mental illness and mental retardation ultimately must be made more profitable than care.

This discussion again addressed the ubiquitous problem in mental health priorities presented by two generations of people in need of mental health services; people already institutionalized and people who will require future institutionalization unless intervention is provided. How should limited resources be divided between these groups? (Where, when, what kind of resources, and provided by whom?) As with other issues, there were no simple answers to this complex question.

The legal concept of "least restrictive alternative" in *Wyatt* has begun to move the locus of legal intervention in the mental health system toward the generation of consumers outside institutions who require less extreme forms of care. In the discussion of a right to treatment, several participants emphasized that the concept should not be restricted to people currently being institutionalized in the mental health system. They asked if a 4-year-old child with Down's Syndrome living at home or a severely depressed parent cared for by his child have the same right to treatment as similar people who are institutionalized. Although strict judicial authority may not extend to these cases, they proposed that a right to treatment needs to focus more broadly on the people residing in the community. Participants viewed inclusion of the large number of potential consumers of mental health services as essential in any effective improvement of the mental health system. When the concept of a right to treatment is expanded to the community, the courts alone are not enough. A set of strategies to attack the system at many fronts was considered necessary for a right to treatment to become more than a dream for the Down's Syndrome child or the depressed parent struggling in the community.

POLITICIZING THE RIGHT TO TREATMENT

The overall strategy needs to include the judiciary as a component and not as a single stroke.

GARRY MARBUT

Judicial intervention has been romantically idealized as a panacea for many social problems, but the federal courts are instruments of intervention only when constitutional issues are raised. Courts can order specific changes to guarantee constitutional rights. However, these courts cannot secure the fiscal or human resources necessary to fulfill the orders without legislative and broader social support. Two decades of frustrated judicial attempts to integrate American public schools were cited to document the dependence of courts upon many other factors to effect meaningful social change. Change in the mental health system in Alabama has been delayed by limited funds arising from an archaic tax structure and the lack of qualified staff willing to work in Alabama. The best efforts by the court, the defendants and plaintiffs cannot alter that situation. The conference participants agreed that other conceptual, political and legislative solutions are necessary to implement adequate care in the mental health system.

Although a right to treatment can be presented to the community on moral or legal grounds, the most persuasive arguments for improvement of the mental health system are economic. Simply stated, custodial care of an individual for 30 years is more expensive than active, intensive treatment for a short time. Furthermore, community treatment is significantly less expensive than institutionalization. Over the last century, the mental health system has amassed large capital investment in antiquated, obsolete institutions and custodial care staffs which have been perpetuated primarily because the political influence of the service providers is greater than the consumers' political influence. As an alternative to the ineffectual, self-serving system, private contracts for specific services were proposed to begin to make human services more manageable and accountable to the consumers' needs. Large capital investments and maintenance costs would not be necessary because facilities such as halfway houses or sheltered workshops could be rented. Program flexibility would be maximized. If the "private sector" entered the mental health system, service providers would become competitive and innovative. A reasonable profit margin for service could attract competent businesses and organizations to provide specific, time-limited services such as staff training, vocation training or job placement for patients.

Within institutions other changes were proposed. Many medical services could be furnished by competent, area professionals on a consultation basis instead of employing full-time professionals who are often semi-invalids, semi-retired or foreign-trained and unqualified to practice medicine. If services were unsatisfactory, the person's contract simply would not be renewed; this is eminently simpler than attempting to remove an incompetent civil service employee. In addition, the use of nonprofessional and paraprofessional persons to supplement staff was suggested as a potential resource for further development.

At a broader level, more general economic incentives were proposed to stimulate change. Although most mental health professionals believe that community care is preferable to institutional care for both the individual and the taxpayers, most states spend the overwhelming parts of their budgets perpetuating institutional treatment. To change this trend, major financial contingencies were suggested to help develop community alternatives. For example, in California the institutionalization of juvenile offenders was dramatically reduced and community facilities were developed by the Short-Doyle Act. This legislation paid counties subsidies to retain and treat their youthful offenders rather than send them to large state institutions. The counties used the money that the state saved by not institutionalizing the youths, to develop more effective community facilities. This significant legislation was not initiated by mental health professionals, but by the state accounting department as an economizing measure that produced major innovation in the human services. Other states could offer counties similar economic incentives to develop local mental health services instead of using large, centralized custodial institutions. Decentralization of human services could also help increase community involvement in planning and monitoring the services.

Others, however, mentioned that many states do not have sufficient funds to provide adequate services for the mentally ill and mentally retarded. The implementation of a federally declared right to treatment may require federal funds (see Mechanic, Chapter 3). Matching fund programs could provide economic incentive to state legislators to invest in improved treatment methods. However, to obtain these resources, participants again emphasized the importance of creating effective political pressure. The central question becomes: Will the necessary political groups be formed to make the right to treatment more than an interesting legal argument?

Even while a right to treatment awaits fulfillment in institutions, the concept of "least restrictive alternative" has expanded legal intervention into other areas of the mental health system. In the absence of clear constitutional issues of deprivation of liberty to justify judicial intervention, participants called for new, imaginative approaches to secure comprehensive changes in the mental health system. Needed, are a new political context and advocate groups for effective human services. Although several national organizations exist, such as the National Association for Mental Health and the American Association for Mental Deficiency, no key group such as the Sierra Club in the ecology movement, exists to publicly focus interest in the mental health field. Instead of single organizations, a coalition of interest groups, mental health professionals, mental health administrators, politicians, legal professionals and consumers were viewed as essential for effective change.

The elusive and difficult task of forming political bridges and coalitions among the divided human service guilds and agencies to improve the delivery of mental health services should begin now. In addition to consolidating professional interests around central goals of improved care, these service-providing groups were urged and warned to begin to be responsive to the consumers of their services. The decades of professional preemption of consumers' prerogatives helped to generate the class action suits brought against institutions and state governments. In the future, consumers of mental health systems and the community are necessary to define goals and form a broad based, political foundation to obtain better human services.

With data on cost effectiveness, not just professional opinion, a well-organized coalition group could effectively lobby to secure more humane services. Politicians respond to political power of organized interest groups. Advocates of a right to treatment agreed that they must learn ways to spark the imagination of the larger community and its leaders. Perhaps labor unions could be courted as allies in securing improved human services. In 1967, the Pennsylvania AFL-CIO gave massive support to the first attempted right-to-treatment legislation. Securing a right to treatment as one component of a right to health would require similar alliances with powerful political groups. In many people's view, mental health professionals have isolated themselves from political processes. Idealistically, assuming that the mental health profession shares the interests of the mental health consumers, that isolation must end if a right to treatment will ever be more than a court order to hire non-existent professional staff with nonappropriated money. Otherwise, this group may become the adversaries instead of the advocates of the mentally ill.

SUMMARY

Decades of neglect of institutionalized citizens and the lack of other interventions have led to a federally declared right to treatment. Questions of the limits of this concept, definitions of mental illness, standards for treatment, the role of the community and the political basis necessary to affect enduring change emerged as central issues in the group discussions of the right to treatment. As one lawyer noted, the right to treatment is a legal neonate, less than a dozen judicial decisions old. As demonstrated by the history of the civil rights movement, social change is often painfully slow. The answers to the many important questions raised by a right to treatment will probably emerge slowly.

Epilog

STUART GOLANN

In the relatively short time since the Amherst Conference several important events have occurred in the definitions of and debate over the right to treatment. Most notable is the development of the cases: *Donaldson v. O'Connor,* now decided by the Supreme Court, and *Wyatt v. Aderholt* (formerly *Wyatt v. Stickney;* Stickney was replaced by Aderholt, who has since been replaced by Hardin).

THE DONALDSON CASE

In a trial that began on November 21, 1972, a Florida jury returned a verdict which awarded Donaldson $28,500 in compensatory damages and $10,000 in punitive damages against O'Connor and Gumanis, who were at different times director of the ward and clinical director of the hospital to which Donaldson had been involuntarily committed in January 1957.

Gumanis and O'Connor separately appealed the decision contending that the Constitution does not guarantee a right to treatment to mental patients involuntarily civilly committed. In part, their appeals were based upon the fact that the trial judge instructed the jury that civilly committed mental patients do have a constitutional right to treatment.

On April 26, 1974, the United States Court of Appeals (Fifth Circuit) in a richly detailed opinion and finding denied both appeals and held that the fourteenth amendment guarantees involuntarily civilly committed mental patients a right to treatment. Note that the *Wyatt v. Aderholt* appeal had been before this same appeals court for two years and that no decision had been forthcoming.

On July 25, 1974, O'Connor petitioned the Supreme Court that a writ of certiorari be issued to review the Appeals Court judgment and opinion. Donaldson's attorneys filed a brief in opposition.

On June 26, 1975, the Supreme Court decided the case, unanimously finding that Donaldson's right to liberty had been violated. Chief Justice Burger issued a separate concurring opinion concerning damages due Donaldson and speculating about the power of states to abridge constitutional rights and the constitutional basis of a related right to treatment.

The Supreme Court decision did not uphold nor did it reverse the Appeals Court findings in *Donaldson* on the right to treatment. Presumably because a new Supreme Court decision (*Wood v. Strickland,* 420 U.S. 308) has clarified the scope of a state official's qualified immunity, the Supreme Court vacated the judgment of the Court of Appeals. Moreover, the Court itself reached no decision of its own on right to treatment:

We have concluded that the difficult issues of constitutional law dealt with by the Court of Appeals are not presented by this case [Donaldson] in its present posture. Specifically, there is no reason now to decide whether mentally ill persons dangerous to themselves or to others have a right to treatment upon compulsory confinement by the State, or whether the State may compulsorily confine a nondangerous, mentally ill individual for the purpose of treatment.

The court did find that

A finding of "mental illness" alone cannot justify a State's locking a person up against his will and keeping him indefinitely in simple custodial confinement. Assuming that that term can be given a reasonably precise content and that the "mentally ill" can be identified with reasonable accuracy, there is still no constitutional basis for confining such persons involuntarily if they are dangerous to no one and can live safely in freedom.

In addition, answering O'Connor's contention that adequacy of treatment is a "nonjusticable" question that must be left to the discretion of the psychiatric profession, the court stated that

Where "treatment" is the sole asserted ground for depriving a person of liberty, it is plainly unacceptable to suggest that the courts are powerless to determine whether the asserted ground is present.

The Decisions of the Court of Appeals and the Supreme Court and Chief Justice Burger's statement are included in the section of Supplementary Case Materials.

THE WYATT CASE

On November 8, 1974, the United States Court of Appeals for the Fifth Circuit handed down a second landmark decision affirming the constitutional right to treatment of persons involuntarily committed to mental institutions. The *Wyatt v. Aderholt* appeal had been before the court for two years. The court unanimously reaffirmed the Alabama District Court decision that there is a right to treatment and specifically rejected the argument that the right cannot be implemented through judicially manageable standards. At the same time the Court reversed the district court decision in *Burnham v. Georgia Department of Public Health.*

Introducing the (now vacated) *Donaldson* decision Judge Wisdom wrote

This case requires us to decide for the first time the far reaching question whether the Fourteenth Amendment guarantees a right to treatment to persons involuntarily civilly committed to state mental hospitals (p. 3131).

In the *Wyatt v. Aderholt* case Judge Wisdom defined the issue in a different way: "In this case," he wrote, "we must decide whether federal district courts have the power to order state mental institutions to provide minimum levels of psychiatric care and treatment to persons civilly committed to the institutions" (p. 715).

Wisdom notes in *Wyatt* that the appellates' (Alabama Mental Health Board and George C. Wallace as Governor) principal contention against a constitutional right to treatment was answered in *Donaldson* where the court held "that civilly committed mental patients have a constitutional right to such individual treatment as will help each of them to be cured or to improve his or her mental condition." Wisdom goes on in the

Wyatt decision to explain the court's reasoning in the *Donaldson* decision:

we reasoned that the only permissible justifications for civil commitment, and for the massive abridgments of constitutionally protected liberties it entails, were the danger posed by the individual's need for treatment and care. We held that where the justification for commitment was treatment, it offended the fundamentals of due process if treatment were not in fact provided; and we held that where the justification was the danger to self or to others, then treatment had to be provided as the quid pro quo society had to pay as the price of the extra safety it derived from the denial of individuals' liberty.

The minimum standards developed for the district court were not challenged in the appeal and, therefore, the appeal court's decision does not rule on them or on the appropriateness of federal court-set standards of state service. Several additional opinions were forthcoming in Wisdom's discussion of *Wyatt*. He denied the state's contention that standard setting invades the legislative preserve because it is linked to appropriation of funds. "It goes without saying," Wisdom said, "that the state legislatures are ordinarily free to choose among various social services competing for legislative attention and state funds. But, that does not mean that a state legislature is free, for budgetary or any other reasons, to provide a social service in a manner which will result in the denial of individuals' constitutional rights."

The difficult questions of the implementation of the right to treatment were remanded back to the district court and Judge Frank Johnson. Wisdom stated that although legislatures can't use the budget to deprive citizens of their rights, there is a "substantial question [as to] the scope of judicial power" in implementing the right to treatment. The court is stating (a) That it can't force a legislature to provide mental hospitals; (b) If a state does provide mental hospitals, the state cannot deprive persons involuntarily civilly committed to their hospitals of constitutional rights on the ground of inadequate funds; (c) That it would be premature for the court to enter into the decision process of how the funds may be obtained. Specifically, the decision says

we regard as premature any issue as to whether the district court should appoint a Special Master for the purpose of selling or encumbering state lands to finance these standards, or should enjoin certain state officials from authorizing expenditures for nonessential state functions, and thereby alter the state budget.

The defendants in *Wyatt* have decided not to take the case any higher and consequently, the *Wyatt* case moves back to the district court for further action on implementation. The most recent action in *Wyatt v. Hardin* concerns the right to refuse treatment. On February 28, 1975, District Court Judge Frank Johnson issued an order modifying Standard 9 of the April 13, 1972 District Court order detailing minimum constitutional requirements for the employment of potentially hazardous modes of treatment. These treatments are "lobotomy, psychosurgery or other unusual, hazardous or intrusive surgical procedure" and "aversive conditioning" or other systematic attempt to modify behavior by means of painful or noxious stimuli. The order resulted in part from action taken by counsel for the plaintiffs when it was learned that some young women at the Partlow School had been sterilized in that institution. Judge Johnson issued standards detailing procedures which must be followed before any resident of the institution is sterilized. The Searcy Human Rights Committee urged the court to provide for greater flexibility in the use of electric convulsive therapy and the court asked the parties and *amici* to propose revisions. The February 28, 1975 order is included among the *Wyatt* supplementary case materials. In addition to *Donaldson* and *Wyatt,* several other important new cases pertain to the rights of hospitalized mentally ill and retarded. Among them are *Welsch et al. v. Likins* and *New York State Association for Retarded Children et al. v. Carey.*

WELSCH V. LIKINS

On February 14, 1974, District Judge Larson decreed that persons civilly committed for reasons of mental retardation "have a right under the due process clause of the Fourteenth Amendment to receive minimally adequate care and treatment . . . and to have defendants explore and seek to provide them with the least restrictive practicable alternatives to hospitalization. . . ." The accompanying memorandum provides another detailed and thoughtful consideration of the constitutional basis of a right to treatment.

NEW YORK STATE ASSOCIATION FOR RETARDED CHILDREN ET AL. V. CAREY (Willowbrook)

On April 30, 1975, a consent decree was signed resolving the two class actions combined into Willowbrook. It included detailed standards for achieving "protection from harm" for the mentally retarded in New York. The decision included provisions for a comprehensive community placement plan to allow Willowbrook to reduce its population drastically along with the establishment of alternative community placements. In addition, the decision called for an individual plan of care, education and training for each of Willowbrook's 3000 current residents to prepare him for life in the community and evaluation by interdisciplinary teams as to the best community alternative for each resident, with no resident placed in the community unless it is determined that the new placement will offer better services and opportunity.

In his accompanying memorandum, Judge Judd noted that "the consent judgment reflects the fact that protection from harm requires relief more extensive than this court originally contemplated, because harm can result not only from neglect but from conditions which cause regression or which prevent development of an individual's capabilities." He wrote further that during the past few years "the fate of the mentally impaired members of our society has passed from an arcane concern to a major issue both of constitutional rights and social policy. . . ."

CASES AND
SOURCE MATERIAL

It should be noted that Wyatt v. Stickney, Wyatt v. Aderholt *and* Wyatt v. Hardin *are all the same case. The changes in the name of the defendant are attributable only to the fact that the Commissioner of Mental Health in Alabama changed several times during the course of the litigation.*

Wyatt v. Stickney

Ricky WYATT, by and through his aunt and legal guardian, Mrs. W. C. Rawlins, Jr., et al., for themselves jointly and severally and for all others similarly situated, Plaintiffs,

v.

Dr. Stonewall B. STICKNEY, as Commissioner of Mental Health and the State of Alabama Mental Health Officer, et al., Defendants,

United States of America et al.,
Amici Curiae.

Civ. A. No. 3195–N.

United States District Court,
M. D. Alabama, N. D.

April 13, 1972.

ORDER AND DECREE

JOHNSON, Chief Judge.

This class action originally was filed on October 23, 1970, in behalf of patients involuntarily confined for mental treatment purposes at Bryce Hospital, Tuscaloosa, Alabama. On March 12, 1971, in a formal opinion and decree, this Court held that these involuntarily committed patients "unquestionably have a constitutional right to receive such individual treatment as will give each of them a realistic opportunity to be cured or to improve his or her mental condition." The Court further held that patients at Bryce were being denied their right to treatment and that defendants, per their request, would be allowed six months in which to raise the level of care at Bryce to the constitutionally required minimum. Wyatt v. Stickney, 325 F.Supp. 781 (M.D.Ala. 1971). In this decree, the Court ordered defendants to file reports defining the mission and functions of Bryce Hospital, specifying the objective and subjective standards required to furnish adequate care to the treatable mentally ill and detailing the hospital's progress toward the implementation of minimum constitutional standards. Subsequent to this order, plaintiffs, by motion to amend granted August 12, 1971, enlarged their class to include patients involuntarily confined for mental treatment at Searcy Hospital [1] and at Partlow State School and Hospital for the mentally retarded. [2]

On September 23, 1971, defendants filed their final report, from which this Court concluded on December 10, 1971, 334 F.Supp. 1341, that defendants had failed to promulgate and implement a treatment program satisfying minimum medical and constitutional requisites. Generally, the Court found that defendants' treatment program was deficient in three fundamental areas. It failed to provide: (1) a humane psychological and physical environment, (2) qualified staff in numbers sufficient to administer adequate treatment and (3) individualized treatment plans. More specifically, the Court found that many conditions, such as nontherapeutic, uncompensated work assignments, and the absence of any semblance of privacy, constituted dehumanizing factors contributing to the degeneration of the patients' self-esteem. The physical facilities at Bryce were overcrowded and plagued by fire and other emergency hazards. The

Court found also that most staff members were poorly trained and that staffing ratios were so inadequate as to render the administration of effective treatment impossible. The Court concluded, therefore, that whatever treatment was provided at Bryce was grossly deficient and failed to satisfy minimum medical and constitutional standards. Based upon this conclusion, the Court ordered that a formal hearing be held at which the parties and amici [3] would have the opportunity to submit proposed standards for constitutionally adequate treatment and to present expert testimony in support of their proposals.

Pursuant to this order, a hearing was held at which the foremost authorities on mental health in the United States appeared and testified as to the minimum medical and constitutional requisites for public institutions, such as Bryce and Searcy, designed to treat the mentally ill. At this hearing, the parties and amici submitted their proposed standards, and now have filed briefs in support of them. [4] Moreover, the parties

1. Searcy Hospital, located in Mount Vernon, Alabama, is also a State institution designed to treat the mentally ill. On September 2, 1971, defendants answered plaintiffs' amended complaint, as it related to Searcy, with the following language:

   "Defendants agree to be bound by the objective and subjective standards ultimately ordered by this Honorable Court in this cause at both Bryce and Searcy."

   This answer obviated the necessity for this Court's holding a formal hearing on the conditions currently existing at Searcy. Nevertheless, the evidence in the record relative to Searcy reflects that the conditions at that institution are no better than those at Bryce.

2. The aspect of the case relating to Partlow State School and Hospital for the mentally retarded will be considered by the Court in a decree separate from the present one.

3. The amici in this case, including the United States of America, the American Orthopsychiatric Association, the American Psychological Association, the American Civil Liberties Union, and the American Association on Mental De-

ficiency, have performed exemplary service for which this Court is indeed grateful.

4. On March 15, 1972, after the hearing in this case, plaintiffs filed a motion for further relief. This motion served, among other things, to renew an earlier motion, filed by plaintiffs on September 1, 1971, and subsequently denied by the Court, to add additional parties. That earlier motion asked that the Court add: "Agnes Baggett, as Treasurer of the State of Alabama; Roy W. Sanders, as Comptroller of the State of Alabama; Ruben King, as Commissioner of the Alabama Department of Pensions and Security, George C. Wallace as Chairman of the Alabama State Board of Pensions and Security, and James J. Bailey as a member of the Alabama State Board of Pensions and Security and as representative of all other members of the Alabama State Board of Pensions and Security; J. Stanley Frazer, as Director of the Alabama State Personnel Board and Ralph W. Adams, as a member of the Alabama State Personnel Board and as representative of all other members of the Alabama State Personnel Board."

and amici have stipulated to a broad spectrum of conditions they feel are mandatory for a constitutionally acceptable minimum treatment program. This Court, having considered the evidence in the case, as well as the briefs, proposed standards and stipulations of the parties, has concluded that the standards set out in Appendix A to this decree are medical and constitutional minimums. Consequently, the Court will order their implementation.[5] In so ordering, however, the Court emphasizes that these standards are, indeed, both medical and constitutional minimums and should be viewed as such. The Court urges that once this order is effectuated, defendants not become complacent and self-satisfied. Rather, they should dedicate themselves to providing physical conditions and treatment programs at Alabama's mental institutions that substantially exceed medical and constitutional minimums.

[1] In addition to asking that their proposed standards be effectuated, plaintiffs and amici have requested other relief designed to guarantee the provision of constitutional and humane treatment. Pursuant to one such request for relief, this Court has determined that it is appropriate to order the initiation of human rights committees to function as standing committees of the Bryce and Searcy facilities. The Court will appoint the members of these committees who shall have review of all research proposals and all rehabilitation programs, to ensure that the dignity and the human rights of patients are preserved. The committees also shall advise and assist patients who allege that their legal rights have been infringed or that the Mental Health Board has failed to comply with judicially ordered guidelines. At their discretion, the committees may consult appropriate, independent specialists who shall be compensated by the defendant Board. Seven members shall comprise the human rights committee for each institution, the names and addresses of whom are set forth in Appendix B to this decree. Those who serve on the committees shall be paid on a per diem basis and be reimbursed for travel expenses at the same rate as members of the Alabama Board of Mental Health.

[2] This Court will reserve ruling upon other forms of relief advocated by plaintiffs and amici, including their prayer for the appointment of a master and a professional advisory committee to oversee the implementation of the

The motion of September 1, 1971, also sought an injunction against the treasurer and the comptroller of the State paying out State funds for "non-essential functions" of the State until enough funds were available to provide adequately for the financial needs of the Alabama State Mental Health Board.

In their motion of March 15, 1972, plaintiffs asked that, in addition to the above-named State officials and agencies, the Court add as parties to this litigation Dr. LeRoy Brown, State Superintendent of Education and Lt. Governor Jere Beasley, State Senator Pierre Pelham and State Representative Sage Lyons, as representatives of the Alabama Legislature. The motion of March 15, 1972, also requested the Court to appoint a master, to appoint a human rights committee and a professional advisory committee, to order the sale of defendant Mental Health Board's land holdings and other assets to raise funds for the operation of Alabama's mental health institutions, to enjoin the construction of any physical facilities by the Mental Health Board and to enjoin the commitment of any more patients to Bryce and Searcy until such time as adequate treatment is supplied in those hospitals.

5. In addition to the standards detailed in this order, it is appropriate that defendants comply also with the conditions, applicable to mental health institutions, necessary to qualify Alabama's facilities for participation in the various programs, such as Medicare and Medicaid, funded by the United States Government. Because many of these conditions of participation have not yet been finally drafted and published, however, this Court will not at this time order that specific Government standards be implemented.

court-ordered minimum constitutional standards.[6] Federal courts are reluctant to assume control of any organization, but especially one operated by a state. This reluctance, combined with defendants' expressed intent that this order will be implemented forthwith and in good faith, causes the Court to withhold its decision on these appointments. Nevertheless, defendants, as well as the other parties and amici in this case, are placed on notice that unless defendants do comply satisfactorily with this order, the Court will be obligated to appoint a master.

[3] Because the availability of financing may bear upon the implementation of this order, the Court is constrained to emphasize at this juncture that a failure by defendants to comply with this decree cannot be justified by a lack of operating funds. As previously established by this Court:

"There can be no legal (or moral) justification for the State of Alabama's failing to afford treatment—and adequate treatment from a medical standpoint—to the several thousand patients who have been civilly committed to Bryce's for treatment purposes. To deprive any citizen of his or her liberty upon the altruistic theory that the confinement is for humane therapeutic reasons and then fail to provide adequate treatment violates the very fundamentals of due process." Wyatt v. Stickney, 325 F.Supp. at 785.

From the above, it follows consistently, of course, that the unavailability of neither funds, nor staff and facilities, will justify a default by defendants in the provision of suitable treatment for the mentally ill.

[4] Despite the possibility that defendants will encounter financial difficulties in the implementation of this order, this Court has decided to reserve ruling also upon plaintiffs' motion that defendant Mental Health Board be directed to sell or encumber portions of its land holdings in order to raise funds.[7] Similarly, this Court will reserve ruling on plaintiffs' motion seeking an injunction against the treasurer and the comptroller of the State authorizing expenditures for nonessential State functions, and on other aspects of plaintiffs' requested relief designed to ameliorate the financial problems incident to the implementation of this order. The Court stresses, however, the extreme importance and the grave immediacy of the need for proper funding of the State's public mental health facilities. The responsibility for appropriate funding ultimately must fall, of course, upon the State Legislature and, to a lesser degree, upon the defendant Mental Health Board of Alabama. For the present time, the Court will defer to those bodies in hopes that they will proceed with the realization and understanding that what is involved in this case is not representative of ordinary governmental functions such as paving roads and maintaining buildings. Rather, what is so inextricably intertwined with how the Legislature and Mental Health Board respond to the revelations of this litigation is the very preservation of human life and dignity. Not only are the lives of the patients currently confined at Bryce and Searcy at stake, but also at issue are the well-

---

6. The Court's decision to reserve its ruling on the appointment of a master necessitates the reservation also of the Court's appointing a professional advisory committee to aid the master. Nevertheless, the Court notes that the professional mental health community in the United States has responded with enthusiasm to the proposed initiation of such a committee to assist in the upgrading of Alabama's mental health facilities. Consequently, this Court strongly recommends to defendants that they develop a professional advisory committee comprised of amenable professionals from throughout the country who are able to provide the expertise the evidence reflects is important to the successful implementation of this order.

7. See n. 4, supra. The evidence presented in this case reflects that the land holdings and other assets of the defendant Board are extensive.

being and security of every citizen of Alabama. As is true in the case of any disease, no one is immune from the peril of mental illness. The problem, therefore, cannot be overemphasized and a prompt response from the Legislature, the Mental Health Board and other responsible State officials, is imperative.

In the event, though, that the Legislature fails to satisfy its well-defined constitutional obligation, and the Mental Health Board, because of lack of funding or any other legally insufficient reason, fails to implement fully the standards herein ordered, it will be necessary for the Court to take affirmative steps, including appointing a master, to ensure that proper funding is realized [8] and that adequate treatment is available for the mentally ill of Alabama.

[5] This Court now must consider that aspect of plaintiffs' motion of March 15, 1972, seeking an injunction against further commitments to Bryce and Searcy until such time as adequate treatment is supplied in those hospitals. Indisputably, the evidence in this case reflects that no treatment program at the Bryce-Searcy facilities approaches constitutional standards. Nevertheless, because of the alternatives to commitment commonly utilized in Alabama, as well as in other states, the Court is fearful that granting plaintiffs' request at the present time would serve only to punish and further deprive Alabama's mentally ill.

[6] Finally, the Court has determined that this case requires the awarding of a reasonable attorneys' fee to plaintiffs' counsel. The basis for the award and the amount thereof will be considered and treated in a separate order. The fee will be charged against

the defendants as a part of the court costs in this case.

To assist the Court in its determination of how to proceed henceforth, defendants will be directed to prepare and file a report within six months from the date of this decree detailing the implementation of each standard herein ordered. This report shall be comprehensive and shall include a statement of the progress made on each standard not yet completely implemented, specifying the reasons for incomplete performance. The report shall include also a statement of the financing secured since the issuance of this decree and of defendants' plans for procuring whatever additional financing might be required. Upon the basis of this report and other available information, the Court will evaluate defendants' work and, in due course, determine the appropriateness of appointing a master and of granting other requested relief.

Accordingly, it is the order, judgment and decree of this Court:

1. That defendants be and they are hereby enjoined from failing to implement fully and with dispatch each of the standards set forth in Appendix A attached hereto and incorporated as a part of this decree;

2. That human rights committees be and are hereby designated and appointed. The members thereof are listed in Appendix B attached hereto and incorporated herein. These committees shall have the purposes, functions, and spheres of operation previously set forth in this order. The members of the committees shall be paid on a per diem basis and be reimbursed for travel expenses at the same rate as members of the Alabama Board of Mental Health;

8. The Court understands and appreciates that the Legislature is not due back in regular session until May, 1973. Nevertheless, special sessions of the Legislature are frequent occurrences in Alabama, and there has never been a time when such a session was more urgently required. If the Legislature does not act promptly to appropriate the necessary funding for mental health, the Court will be compelled to grant plaintiffs' motion to add various State officials and agencies as additional parties to this litigation, and to utilize other avenues of fund raising.

3. That defendants, within six months from this date, prepare and file with this Court a report reflecting in detail the progress on the implementation of this order. This report shall be comprehensive and precise, and shall explain the reasons for incomplete performance in the event the defendants have not met a standard in its entirety. The report also shall include a financial statement and an up-to-date timetable for full compliance.

4. That the court costs incurred in this proceeding, including a reasonable attorneys' fee for plaintiffs' lawyers, be and they are hereby taxed against the defendants;

5. That jurisdiction of this cause be and the same is hereby specifically retained.

It is further ordered that ruling on plaintiffs' motion for further relief, including the appointment of a master, filed March 15, 1972, be and the same is hereby reserved.

APPENDIX A

MINIMUM CONSTITUTIONAL STANDARDS FOR ADEQUATE TREATMENT OF THE MENTALLY ILL

I. *Definitions*:

a. "Hospital"—Bryce and Searcy Hospitals.

b. "Patients"—all persons who are now confined and all persons who may in the future be confined at Bryce and Searcy Hospitals pursuant to an involuntary civil commitment procedure.

c. "Qualified Mental Health Professional"—

(1) a psychiatrist with three years of residency training in psychiatry;

(2) a psychologist with a doctoral degree from an accredited program;

(3) a social worker with a master's degree from an accredited program and two years of clinical experience under the supervision of a Qualified Mental Health Professional;

(4) a registered nurse with a graduate degree in psychiatric nursing and two years of clinical experience under the supervision of a Qualified Mental Health Professional.

d. "Non-Professional Staff Member" —an employee of the hospital, other than a Qualified Mental Health Professional, whose duties require contact with or supervision of patients.

II. *Humane Psychological and Physical Environment*

1. Patients have a right to privacy and dignity.

2. Patients have a right to the least restrictive conditions necessary to achieve the purposes of commitment.

3. No person shall be deemed incompetent to manage his affairs, to contract, to hold professional or occupational or vehicle operator's licenses, to marry and obtain a divorce, to register and vote, or to make a will *solely* by reason of his admission or commitment to the hospital.

4. Patients shall have the same rights to visitation and telephone communications as patients at other public hospitals, except to the extent that the Qualified Mental Health Professional responsible for formulation of a particular patient's treatment plan writes an order imposing special restrictions. The written order must be renewed after each periodic review of the treatment plan if any restrictions are to be continued. Patients shall have an unrestricted right to visitation with attorneys and with private physicians and other health professionals.

5. Patients shall have an unrestricted right to send sealed mail. Patients shall have an unrestricted right to receive sealed mail from their attorneys, private physicians, and other mental health professionals, from courts, and government officials. Patients shall have a right to receive sealed mail from others, except to the extent that the Qualified Mental Health Professional responsible for formulation of a particular

patient's treatment plan writes an order imposing special restrictions on receipt of sealed mail. The written order must be renewed after each periodic review of the treatment plan if any restrictions are to be continued.

6. Patients have a right to be free from unnecessary or excessive medication. No medication shall be administered unless at the written order of a physician. The superintendent of the hospital and the attending physician shall be responsible for all medication given or administered to a patient. The use of medication shall not exceed standards of use that are advocated by the United States Food and Drug Administration. Notation of each individual's medication shall be kept in his medical records. At least weekly the attending physician shall review the drug regimen of each patient under his care. All prescriptions shall be written with a termination date, which shall not exceed 30 days. Medication shall not be used as punishment, for the convenience of staff, as a substitute for program, or in quantities that interfere with the patient's treatment program.

7. Patients have a right to be free from physical restraint and isolation. Except for emergency situations, in which it is likely that patients could harm themselves or others and in which less restrictive means of restraint are not feasible, patients may be physically restrained or placed in isolation only on a Qualified Mental Health Professional's written order which explains the rationale for such action. The written order may be entered only after the Qualified Mental Health Professional has personally seen the patient concerned and evaluated whatever episode or situation is said to call for restraint or isolation. Emergency use of restraints or isolation shall be for no more than one hour, by which time a Qualified Mental Health Professional shall have been consulted and shall have entered an appropriate order in writing. Such written order shall be effective for no more than 24 hours and must be renewed if restraint and isolation are to be continued. While

in restraint or isolation the patient must be seen by qualified ward personnel who will chart the patient's physical condition (if it is compromised) and psychiatric condition every hour. The patient must have bathroom privileges every hour and must be bathed every 12 hours.

8. Patients shall have a right not to be subjected to experimental research without the express and informed consent of the patient, if the patient is able to give such consent, and of his guardian or next of kin, after opportunities for consultation with independent specialists and with legal counsel. Such proposed research shall first have been reviewed and approved by the institution's Human Rights Committee before such consent shall be sought. Prior to such approval the Committee shall determine that such research complies with the principles of the Statement on the Use of Human Subjects for Research of the American Association on Mental Deficiency and with the principles for research involving human subjects required by the United States Department of Health, Education and Welfare for projects supported by that agency.

9. Patients have a right not to be subjected to treatment procedures such as lobotomy, electro-convulsive treatment, adversive reinforcement conditioning or other unusual or hazardous treatment procedures without their express and informed consent after consultation with counsel or interested party of the patient's choice.

10. Patients have a right to receive prompt and adequate medical treatment for any physical ailments.

11. Patients have a right to wear their own clothes and to keep and use their own personal possessions except insofar as such clothes or personal possessions may be determined by a Qualified Mental Health Professional to be dangerous or otherwise inappropriate to the treatment regimen.

12. The hospital has an obligation to supply an adequate allowance of clothing to any patients who do not have suitable clothing of their own. Patients shall

have the opportunity to select from various types of neat, clean, and seasonable clothing. Such clothing shall be considered the patient's throughout his stay in the hospital.

13. The hospital shall make provision for the laundering of patient clothing.

14. Patients have a right to regular physical exercise several times a week. Moreover, it shall be the duty of the hospital to provide facilities and equipment for such exercise.

15. Patients have a right to be outdoors at regular and frequent intervals, in the absence of medical considerations.

16. The right to religious worship shall be accorded to each patient who desires such opportunities. Provisions for such worship shall be made available to all patients on a nondiscriminatory basis. No individual shall be coerced into engaging in any religious activities.

17. The institution shall provide, with adequate supervision, suitable opportunities for the patient's interaction with members of the opposite sex.

18. The following rules shall govern patient labor:

A. *Hospital Maintenance* No patient shall be required to perform labor which involves the operation and maintenance of the hospital or for which the hospital is under contract with an outside organization. Privileges or release from the hospital shall not be conditioned upon the performance of labor covered by this provision. Patients may voluntarily engage in such labor if the labor is compensated in accordance with the minimum wage laws of the Fair Labor Standards Act, 29 U.S.C. § 206 as amended, 1966.

B. *Therapeutic Tasks and Therapeutic Labor*

(1) Patients may be required to perform therapeutic tasks which do not involve the operation and maintenance of the hospital, provided the specific task or any change in assignment is:

    a. An integrated part of the patient's treatment plan and approved as a therapeutic activity by a Qualified Mental Health Professional responsible for supervising the patient's treatment; and

    b. Supervised by a staff member to oversee the therapeutic aspects of the activity.

(2) Patients may voluntarily engage in therapeutic labor for which the hospital would otherwise have to pay an employee, provided the specific labor or any change in labor assignment is:

    a. An integrated part of the patient's treatment plan and approved as a therapeutic activity by a Qualified Mental Health Professional responsible for supervising the patient's treatment; and

    b. Supervised by a staff member to oversee the therapeutic aspects of the activity; and

    c. Compensated in accordance with the minimum wage laws of the Fair Labor Standards Act, 29 U.S.C. § 206 as amended, 1966.

C. *Personal Housekeeping* Patients may be required to perform tasks of a personal housekeeping nature such as the making of one's own bed.

D. Payment to patients pursuant to these paragraphs shall not be applied to the costs of hospitalization.

19. *Physical Facilities*

A patient has a right to a humane psychological and physical environment within the hospital facilities. These facilities shall be designed to afford patients with comfort and safety, promote dignity, and ensure privacy. The facilities shall be designed to make a positive contribution to the efficient attainment of the treatment goals of the hospital.

A. *Resident Unit*

The number of patients in a multi-patient room shall not exceed six persons. There shall be allocated a minimum of 80 square feet of floor space per patient in a multi-patient room. Screens or curtains shall be provided to ensure privacy within the resident unit. Single rooms shall have a minimum of 100 square feet of floor space. Each patient will be furnished with a comfortable bed with adequate changes of linen, a closet or locker for his personal belongings, a chair, and a bedside table.

B. *Toilets and Lavatories*

There will be one toilet provided for each eight patients and one lavatory for each six patients. A lavatory will be provided with each toilet facility. The toilets will be installed in separate stalls to ensure privacy, will be clean and free of odor, and will be equipped with appropriate safety devices for the physically handicapped.

C. *Showers*

There will be one tub or shower for each 15 patients. If a central bathing area is provided, each shower area will be divided by curtains to ensure privacy. Showers and tubs will be equipped with adequate safety accessories.

D. *Day Room*

The minimum day room area shall be 40 square feet per patient. Day rooms will be attractive and adequately furnished with reading lamps, tables, chairs, television and other recreational facilities. They will be conveniently located to patients' bedrooms and shall have outside windows. There shall be at least one day room area on each bedroom floor in a multi-story hospital. Areas used for corridor traffic cannot be counted as day room space; nor can a chapel with fixed pews be counted as a day room area.

E. *Dining Facilities*

The minimum dining room area shall be ten square feet per patient. The dining room shall be separate from the kitchen and will be furnished with comfortable chairs and tables with hard, washable surfaces.

F. *Linen Servicing and Handling*

The hospital shall provide adequate facilities and equipment for handling clean and soiled bedding and other linen. There must be frequent changes of bedding and other linen, no less than every seven days to assure patient comfort.

G. *Housekeeping*

Regular housekeeping and maintenance procedures which will ensure that the hospital is maintained in a safe, clean, and attractive condition will be developed and implemented.

H. *Geriatric and Other Nonambulatory Mental Patients*

There must be special facilities for geriatric and other nonambulatory patients to assure their safety and comfort, including special fittings on toilets and wheelchairs. Appropriate provision shall be made to permit nonambulatory patients to communicate their needs to staff.

I. *Physical Plant*

(1) Pursuant to an established routine maintenance and repair program, the physical plant shall be kept in a continuous state of good repair and operation in accordance with the needs of the health, comfort, safety and well-being of the patients.

(2) Adequate heating, air conditioning and ventilation systems and equipment shall be afforded to maintain temperatures and air changes which are required for the comfort of patients at all times and the removal of undesired heat, steam and offensive odors. Such facilities shall ensure that the temperature in the hospital shall not exceed 83°F nor fall below 68°F.

(3) Thermostatically controlled hot water shall be provided in adequate quantities and maintained at the required temperature for patient or resident use (110°F at the fixture) and for mechanical dishwashing and laundry use (180°F at the equipment).

(4) Adequate refuse facilities will be provided so that solid waste, rubbish and other refuse will be collected and disposed of in a manner which will prohibit transmission of disease and not create a nuisance or fire hazard or provide a breeding place for rodents and insects.

(5) The physical facilities must meet all fire and safety standards established

by the state and locality. In addition, the hospital shall meet such provisions of the Life Safety Code of the National Fire Protection Association (21st edition, 1967) as are applicable to hospitals.

19A. The hospital shall meet all standards established by the state for general hospitals, insofar as they are relevant to psychiatric facilities.

20. *Nutritional Standards*

Patients, except for the non-mobile, shall eat or be fed in dining rooms. The diet for patients will provide at a minimum the Recommended Daily Dietary Allowances as developed by the National Academy of Sciences. Menus shall be satisfying and nutritionally adequate to provide the Recommended Daily Dietary Allowances. In developing such menus, the hospital will utilize the Low Cost Food Plan of the Department of Agriculture. The hospital will not spend less per patient for raw food, including the value of donated food, than the most recent per person costs of the Low Cost Food Plan for the Southern Region of the United States, as compiled by the United States Department of Agriculture, for appropriate groupings of patients, discounted for any savings which might result from institutional procurement of such food. Provisions shall be made for special therapeutic diets and for substitutes at the request of the patient, or his guardian or next of kin, in accordance with the religious requirements of any patient's faith. Denial of a nutritionally adequate diet shall not be used as punishment.

III. *Qualified Staff in Numbers Sufficient to Administer Adequate Treatment*

21. Each Qualified Mental Health Professional shall meet all licensing and certification requirements promulgated by the State of Alabama for persons engaged in private practice of the same profession elsewhere in Alabama. Other staff members shall meet the same licensing and certification requirements as persons who engage in private practice of their speciality elsewhere in Alabama.

22. a. All Non-Professional Staff Members who have not had prior clinical experience in a mental institution shall have a substantial orientation training.

   b. Staff members on all levels shall have regularly scheduled in-service training.

23. Each Non-Professional Staff Member shall be under the direct supervision of a Qualified Mental Health Professional.

24. *Staffing Ratios*

The hospital shall have the following minimum numbers of treatment personnel per 250 patients. Qualified Mental Health Professionals trained in particular disciplines may in appropriate situations perform services or functions traditionally performed by members of other disciplines. Changes in staff deployment may be made with prior approval of this Court upon a clear and convincing demonstration that the proposed deviation from this staffing structure will enhance the treatment of the patients.

Classification	Number of Employees
Unit Director	1
Psychiatrist (3 years' residency training in psychiatry)	2
MD (Registered physicians)	4
Nurses (RN)	12
Licensed Practical Nurses	6
Aide III	6
Aide II	16
Aide I	70
Hospital Orderly	10
Clerk Stenographer II	3
Clerk Typist II	3
Unit Administrator	1
Administrative Clerk	1
Psychologist (Ph.D.) (doctoral degree from accredited program)	1
Psychologist (M.A.)	1
Psychologist (B.S.)	2
Social Worker (MSW) (from accredited program)	2
Social Worker (B.A.)	5
Patient Activity Therapist (M.S.)	1
Patient Activity Aide	10
Mental Health Technician	10
Dental Hygienist	1

Classification	Number of Employees
Chaplain	.5
Vocational Rehabilitation Counselor	1
Volunteer Services Worker	1
Mental Health Field Representative	1
Dietitian	1
Food Service Supervisor	1
Cook II	2
Cook I	3
Food Service Worker	15
Vehicle Driver	1
Housekeeper	10
Messenger	1
Maintenance Repairman	2

IV. *Individualized Treatment Plans*

25. Each patient shall have a comprehensive physical and mental examination and review of behavioral status within 48 hours after admission to the hospital.

26. Each patient shall have an individualized treatment plan. This plan shall be developed by appropriate Qualified Mental Health Professionals, including a psychiatrist, and implemented as soon as possible—in any event no later than five days after the patient's admission. Each individualized treatment plan shall contain:

   a. a statement of the nature of the specific problems and specific needs of the patient;

   b. a statement of the least restrictive treatment conditions necessary to achieve the purposes of commitment;

   c. a description of intermediate and long-range treatment goals, with a projected timetable for their attainment;

   d. a statement and rationale for the plan of treatment for achieving these intermediate and long-range goals;

   e. a specification of staff responsibility and a description of proposed staff involvement with the patient in order to attain these treatment goals;

   f. criteria for release to less restrictive treatment conditions, and criteria for discharge;

   g. a notation of any therapeutic tasks and labor to be performed by the patient in accordance with Standard 18.

27. As part of his treatment plan, each patient shall have an individualized post-hospitalization plan. This plan shall be developed by a Qualified Mental Health Professional as soon as practicable after the patient's admission to the hospital.

28. In the interests of continuity of care, whenever possible, one Qualified Mental Health Professional (who need not have been involved with the development of the treatment plan) shall be responsible for supervising the implementation of the treatment plan, integrating the various aspects of the treatment program and recording the patient's progress. This Qualified Mental Health Professional shall also be responsible for ensuring that the patient is released, where appropriate, into a less restrictive form of treatment.

29. The treatment plan shall be continuously reviewed by the Qualified Mental Health Professional responsible for supervising the implementation of the plan and shall be modified if necessary. Moreover, at least every 90 days, each patient shall receive a mental examination from, and his treatment plan shall be reviewed by, a Qualified Mental Health Professional other than the professional responsible for supervising the implementation of the plan.

30. In addition to treatment for mental disorders, patients confined at mental health institutions also are entitled to and shall receive appropriate treatment for physical illnesses such as tuberculosis.[1] In providing medical care, the State Board of Mental Health shall take advantage of whatever community-based facilities are appropriate and available and shall coordinate the patient's treatment for mental illness with his medical treatment.

---

1. Approximately 50 patients at Bryce-Searcy are tubercular as also are approximately four residents at Partlon.

31. Complete patient records shall be kept on the ward in which the patient is placed and shall be available to anyone properly authorized in writing by the patient. These records shall include:

a. Identification data, including the patient's legal status;

b. A patient history, including but not limited to:

(1) family data, educational background, and employment record;

(2) prior medical history, both physical and mental, including prior hospitalization;

c. The chief complaints of the patient and the chief complaints of others regarding the patient;

d. An evaluation which notes the onset of illness, the circumstances leading to admission, attitudes, behavior, estimate of intellectual functioning, memory functioning, orientation, and an inventory of the patient's assets in descriptive, not interpretative, fashion;

e. A summary of each physical examination which describes the results of the examination;

f. A copy of the individual treatment plan and any modifications thereto;

g. A detailed summary of the findings made by the reviewing Qualified Mental Health Professional after each periodic review of the treatment plan which analyzes the successes and failures of the treatment program and directs whatever modifications are necessary;

h. A copy of the individualized posthospitalization plan and any modifications thereto, and a summary of the steps that have been taken to implement that plan;

i. A medication history and status, which includes the signed orders of the prescribing physician. Nurses shall indicate by signature that orders have been carried out;

j. A detailed summary of each significant contact by a Qualified Mental Health Professional with the patient;

k. A detailed summary on at least a weekly basis by a Qualified Mental Health Professional involved in the patient's treatment of the patient's progress along the treatment plan;

l. A weekly summary of the extent and nature of the patient's work activities described in Standard 18, *supra,* and the effect of such activity upon the patient's progress along the treatment plan;

m. A signed order by a Qualified Mental Health Professional for any restrictions on visitations and communication, as provided in Standards 4 and 5, *supra;*

n. A signed order by a Qualified Mental Health Professional for any physical restraints and isolation, as provided in Standard 7, *supra;*

o. A detailed summary of any extraordinary incident in the hospital involving the patient to be entered by a staff member noting that he has personal knowledge of the incident or specifying his other source of information, and initialed within 24 hours by a Qualified Mental Health Professional;

p. A summary by the superintendent of the hospital or his appointed agent of his findings after the 15-day review provided for in Standard 33 *infra.*

32. In addition to complying with all the other standards herein, a hospital shall make special provisions for the treatment of patients who are children and young adults. These provisions shall include but are not limited to:

a. Opportunities for publicly supported education suitable to the educational needs of the patient. This program of education must, in the opinion of the attending Qualified Mental Health Professional, be compatible with the patient's mental condition and his treatment program, and otherwise be in the patient's best interest.

b. A treatment plan which considers the chronological, maturational, and developmental level of the patient;

c. Sufficient Qualified Mental Health Professionals, teachers, and staff members with specialized skills in the care and treatment of children and young adults;

d. Recreation and play opportunities in the open air where possible and appropriate residential facilities;

e. Arrangements for contact between the hospital and the family of the patient.

33. No later than 15 days after a patient is committed to the hospital, the superintendent of the hospital or his appointed, professionally qualified agent shall examine the committed patient and shall determine whether the patient continues to require hospitalization and whether a treatment plan complying with Standard 26 has been implemented. If the patient no longer requires hospitalization in accordance with the standards for commitment, or if a treatment plan has not been implemented, he must be released immediately unless he agrees to continue with treatment on a voluntary basis.

34. The Mental Health Board and its agents have an affirmative duty to provide adequate transitional treatment and care for all patients released after a period of involuntary confinement. Transitional care and treatment possibilities include, but are not limited to, psychiatric day care, treatment in the home by a visiting therapist, nursing home or extended care, out-patient treatment, and treatment in the psychiatric ward of a general hospital.

V. *Miscellaneous*

35. Each patient and his family, guardian, or next friend shall promptly upon the patient's admission receive written notice, in language he understands, of all the above standards for adequate treatment. In addition a copy of all the above standards shall be posted in each ward.

APPENDIX B

BRYCE HUMAN RIGHTS COMMITTEE

1. Mr. Bert Bank—Chairman — P. O. Box 2149, Tuscaloosa, Alabama 35401
2. Ms. Ruth Cummings Bolden — 1414 9th Street, Tuscaloosa, Alabama 35401
3. Ms. Babs Klein Heilpern — 2526 Jasmine Road, Montgomery, Alabama 36111
4. Mr. Joseph Mallisham — 3028 20th Street, Tuscaloosa, Alabama 35401
5. Ms. Alberta Murphy — 13 Hillcrest, Tuscaloosa, Alabama 35401
6. Mr. Junior Richardson — 17 CW, Bryce Hospital, Tuscaloosa, Alabama 35401
7. Mr. John T. Wagnon, Jr. — 822 Felder Avenue, Montgomery, Alabama 36106

SEARCY HUMAN RIGHTS COMMITTEE

1. Dr. E. L. McCafferty, Jr.—Chairman — 1653 Spring Hill Avenue, Mobile, Alabama 36604
2. Hon. James U. Blacksher — 304 South Monterey, Mobile, Alabama
3. Hon. Thomas E. Gilmore — P. O. Box 109, Eutaw, Alabama 35462
4. Ms. Consuello J. Harper — 3114 Caffey Drive, Montgomery, Alabama 36108
5. Hon. Horace McCloud — Mount Vernon, Alabama
6. Sister Eileen McLoughlin — 404 Government Street, Mobile, Alabama 36601
7. Ms. Joyce Nickels — c/o Searcy Hospital, Mount Vernon, Alabama

Ricky WYATT, by and through his aunt and legal guardian, Mrs. W. C. Rawlins, Jr., et al., for themselves jointly and severally and for all others similarly situated, Plaintiffs,

v.

Dr. Stonewall B. STICKNEY, as Commissioner of Mental Health and the State of Alabama Mental Health Officer, et al., Defendants,

United States of America et al., Amici Curiae.

Civ. A. No. 3195–N.

United States District Court,
M. D. Alabama, N. D.

April 13, 1972.

Attorneys' Fees Taxed June 2, 1972.

ORDER AND DECREE

JOHNSON, Chief Judge.

This litigation originally pertained only to Alabama's mentally ill,[1] but by motion to amend granted August 12, 1971, plaintiffs have expanded their class to include residents of Partlow State School and Hospital, a public institution located in Tuscaloosa, Alabama, designed to habilitate the mentally retarded.[2] In their amended complaint, plaintiffs have

1. On March 12, 1971, in a formal opinion and decree, this Court held that patients involuntarily committed to Bryce Hospital because of mental illness were being deprived of the constitutional right, which they unquestionably possess, "to receive such individual treatment as [would] give each of them a realistic opportunity to be cured or to improve his or her mental condition." Wyatt v. Stickney, 325 F.Supp. 781 (M.D.Ala.1971). On August 12, 1971, the Court granted plaintiffs' motion to add to the lawsuit patients confined at Searcy Hospital, Mount Vernon, Alabama, another institution which, although designed to treat the mentally ill, failed to do so in accordance with constitutional standards. The Court, having unavailingly afforded defendants an opportunity to promulgate and effectuate minimum standards for adequate treatment of the mentally ill, determined on December 10, 1971, that such standards had to be judicially formulated and ordered implemented. Wyatt v. Stickney, 334 F.Supp. 1341 (M.D.Ala.1971). To that end, the Court conducted a hearing on February 3–4, 1972, at which the parties and amici submitted proposed standards for constitutionally adequate treatment, and presented expert testimony in support of the proposals. The aspect of

alleged that Partlow is being operated in a constitutionally impermissible fashion and that, as a result, its residents are denied the right to adequate habilitation. Relying on these allegations, plaintiffs have asked that the Court promulgate and order the implementation at Partlow of minimum medical and constitutional standards appropriate for the functioning of such an institution. Plaintiffs have asked also that the Court appoint a master and a professional advisory committee to oversee the implementation of judicially ordered guidelines and appoint a human rights committee to safeguard the personal rights and dignity of the residents. Finally plaintiffs have requested the Court to grant various forms of relief intended to ameliorate the financial difficulties certain to arise in connection with the upgrading of Alabama's public mental health institutions.[3]

the case relating to the Bryce-Searcy facilities will be considered by the Court in a decree separate from the present one.

2. As expressed by amici in their briefs and substantiated by the evidence in this case, *mental retardation* refers generally to subaverage intellectual functioning which is associated with impairment in adaptive behavior. This definitional approach to mental retardation is based upon dual criteria: reduced intellectual functioning and impairment in adaptation to the requirements of social living. The evidence presented reflects scientific advances in understanding the developmental processes of the mental retardate. The historic view of mental retardation as an immutable defect of intelligence has been supplanted by the recognition that a person may be mentally retarded at one age level and not at another; that he may change status as a result of changes in the level of his intellectual functioning; or that he may move from retarded to nonretarded as a result of a training program which has increased his level of adaptive behavior to a point where his behavior is no longer of concern to society. See United States President's Panel on Mental Retardation, Report of the Task Force on Law, 1963. (Judge David L. Bazelon, Chairman.)

3. More specifically, in a motion filed September 1, 1971, and renewed March 15, 1972, plaintiffs have asked that they be permitted to join various state officials as defendants in this case. Plaintiffs

On February 28–29, 1972, the Court conducted a hearing on the issues formulated by the pleadings in this case. Evidence was taken on the adequacy of conditions currently existing at Partlow as well as on the standards requisite for a constitutionally acceptable minimum habilitation program. The parties and amici [4] stipulated to a broad array of these standards and proposed additional ones for the Court's evaluation. The case now is submitted upon the pleadings, the evidence, the stipulations, and the proposed standards and briefs of the parties.

[1] Initially, this Court has considered plaintiffs' position, not actively contested by defendants, that people involuntarily committed [5] through noncriminal procedures to institutions for the mentally retarded have a constitutional right to receive such individual habilitation as will give each of them a realistic opportunity to lead a more useful and meaningful life and to return to society. That this position is in accord with the applicable legal principles is clear beyond cavil. In an analogous situation involving the mentally ill at Bryce Hospital, this Court said:

> "Adequate and effective treatment is constitutionally required because, absent treatment, the hospital is transformed 'into a penitentiary where one could be held indefinitely for no convicted offense.' Ragsdale v. Overholser, [108 U.S.App.D.C. 308] 281 F.2d 943, 950 (1960). The purpose of involuntary hospitalization for treatment purposes is *treatment* and not mere custodial care or punishment. This is the only justification, from a constitutional standpoint, that allows civil commitments to mental institutions such as Bryce." Wyatt v. Stickney, 325 F.Supp. at 784.

In the context of the right to appropriate care for people civilly confined to public mental institutions, no viable distinction can be made between the mentally ill and the mentally retarded. Because the only constitutional justification for civilly committing a mental retardate, therefore, is habilitation, it follows ineluctably that once committed such a person is possessed of an inviolable constitutional right to habilitation.[6]

---

maintain that these officials, including, among others, the members of the State Legislature and the treasurer and the comptroller of Alabama, are necessary parties for the attainment of complete relief. Among the relief plaintiffs seek in connection with the state officials is an injunction against the expenditure of state funds for nonessential functions of the state until enough money is available to provide adequately for the financial needs of the Alabama Mental Health Board. In addition, plaintiffs have asked the Court to order the sale of a portion of defendant Mental Health Board's land holdings and other assets and to enjoin the Board from the construction of any physical facilities, including any planned for regional centers.

4. The amici in this case, including the United States of America, the American Orthopsychiatric Association, the American Psychological Association, the American Civil Liberties Union, and the American Association on Mental Deficiency, have performed invaluable service for which this Court is indeed appreciative.

5. The Court will deal in this decree only with residents involuntarily committed to Partlow because no evidence has been adduced tending to demonstrate that any resident is voluntarily confined in that institution. The Court will presume, therefore, that every resident of Partlow is entitled to constitutionally minimum habilitation. The burden falls squarely upon the institution to prove that a particular resident has not been involuntarily committed, and only if defendants satisfy this difficult burden of proof will the Court be confronted with whether the voluntarily committed resident has a right to habilitation.

6. It is interesting to note that the Court's decision with regard to the right of the mentally retarded to habilitation is supported not only by applicable legal authority, but also by a resolution adopted on December 27, 1971, by the General Assembly of the United Nations. That resolution, entitled "Declaration on the Rights of the Mentally Retarded", reads in pertinent part:

Having recognized the existence of this right, the Court now must determine whether prevailing conditions at Partlow conform to minimum standards constitutionally required for a mental retardation institution. The Court's conclusion, compelled by the evidence, is unmistakably clear. Put simply, conditions at Partlow are grossly substandard. Testimony presented by plaintiffs and amici has depicted hazardous and deplorable inadequacies in the institution's operation.[7] Commendably, defendants have offered no rebuttal.[8] At the close of the testimony, the Court, having been impressed by the urgency of the situation, issued an interim emergency order "to protect the lives and well-being of the residents of Partlow." In that order, the Court found that:

"The evidence . . . has vividly and undisputedly portrayed Partlow State School and Hospital as a warehousing institution which, because of its atmosphere of psychological and physical deprivation, is wholly incapable of furnishing [habilitation] to the mentally retarded and is conducive only to the deterioration and the debilitation of the residents. The evidence has reflected further that safety and sanitary conditions at Partlow are substandard to the point of endangering the health and lives of those residing there, that the wards are grossly understaffed, rendering even simple custodial care impossible, and that overcrowding remains a dangerous problem often leading to serious accidents, some of which have resulted in deaths of residents." Wyatt v. Stickney, March 2, 1972. (Unreported Interim Emergency Order.)

[2] Based upon these findings, the Court has concluded that plaintiffs have been denied their right to habilitation and that, pursuant to plaintiffs' request, minimum standards for constitutional care and training must be effectuated at Partlow. Consequently, having determined from a careful study of the evi-

---

". . . The mentally retarded person has a right to proper medical care and physical therapy and to such education, training, rehabilitation and guidance as will enable him to develop his ability and maximum potential."

7. The most comprehensive testimony on the conditions currently prevailing at Partlow was elicited from Dr. Philip Roos, the Executive Director of the National Association for Retarded Children. Dr. Roos inspected Partlow over a two-day period and testified as to his subjective evaluation of the institution. In concluding his testimony, Dr. Roos summarized as follows:

" . . . I feel that the institution and its programs as now conceived are incapable of providing habilitation of the residents. Incarceration, certainly for most of the residents, would I feel have adverse consequences; would tend to develop behaviors which would interfere with successful community functioning. I would anticipate to find stagnation or deterioration in physical, intellectual, and social spheres. The conditions at Partlow today are generally dehumanizing, fostering deviancy, generating self-fulfilling prophecy of parasitism and helplessness. The conditions I would say are hazardous to psychologi-

cal integrity, to health, and in some cases even to life. The administration, the physical plants, the programs, and the institution's articulation with the community and with the consumers reflect destructive models of mental retardation. They hark back to decades ago when the retarded were misperceived as being sick, as being threats to society, or as being subhuman organisms. The new concepts in the field of mental retardation are unfortunately not reflected in Partlow as we see it today—concepts such as normalization, developmental model in orientation toward mental retardation, the thrust of consumer involvement, the trend toward community orientation and decentralization of services; none of these are clearly in evidence in the facility today."

8. Indeed, on February 22, 1972, defendants filed with the Court a statement of position providing in relevant part that:
"Assuming that such a federal constitutional obligation exists . . . ., defendants will not contest the factual accuracy of an ultimate finding . . . that defendants have not met the constitutional obligation to provide adequate care at [Partlow], . . ."
At the hearing, defendants adopted the testimony of Dr. Roos in its entirety.

dence that the standards set out in Appendix A to this decree are medical and constitutional minimums, this Court will order their implementation.[9] In so ordering, the Court emphasizes that these standards are, indeed, minimums only peripherally approaching the ideal to which defendants should aspire. It is hoped that the revelations of this case will furnish impetus to defendants to provide physical facilities and habilitation programs at Partlow substantially exceeding medical and constitutional minimums.

[3] For the present, however, defendants must realize that the prompt institution of minimum standards to ensure the provision of essential care and training for Alabama's mental retardates is mandatory and that no default can be justified by a want of operating funds. In this regard, the principles applicable to the mentally ill apply with equal force to the mentally retarded. See Wyatt v. Stickney, 325 F.Supp. at 784–785.

[4] In addition to requesting that minimum standards be implemented, plaintiffs have asked that defendants be directed to establish a standing human rights committee to guarantee that residents are afforded constitutional and humane habilitation. The evidence reflects that such a committee is needed at Partlow, and this Court will order its initiation. This committee shall have review of all research proposals and all habilitation programs to ensure that the dignity and human rights of residents

are preserved. The committee also shall advise and assist residents who allege that their legal rights have been infringed or that the Mental Health Board has failed to comply with judicially ordered guidelines. At reasonable times the committee may inspect the records of the institution and interview residents and staff. At its discretion the committee may consult appropriate, independent specialists who shall be compensated by the defendant Board.[10] The Court will appoint seven members to comprise Partlow's human rights committee, the names and addresses of whom are set forth in Appendix B to this decree. Those who serve on the committee shall be paid on a per diem basis and be reimbursed for travel expenses at the same rate as members of the Alabama Board of Mental Health.

[5] Plaintiffs, as well as amici, also have advocated the appointment of a federal master and a professional advisory committee to oversee the implementation of minimum constitutional standards. These parties maintain that conditions at Partlow largely are the product of shameful neglect by the state officials charged with responsibility for that institution. Consequently, plaintiffs and amici insist, these state officials have proved themselves incapable of instituting a constitutional habilitation program. Although this Court acknowledges the intolerable conditions at Partlow and recognizes defendants' past nonfeasances, it, nevertheless, reserves ruling on the appointment of a master and a professional advisory committee.[11] Fed-

---

9. In addition to the standards detailed in this order, it is appropriate that defendants comply also with the conditions, applicable to mental health institutions, necessary to qualify Partlow for participation in the various programs, such as Medicare and Medicaid, funded by the United States Government. Because many of these conditions of participation have not yet been finally drafted and published, however, this Court will not at this time order that specific Government standards be implemented.

10. The recitation of the licenses of this committee, and similarly, of the com-

mittees to be inaugurated at the Bryce and Searcy facilities, is not intended to be inclusive. The human rights committee of each mental health institution shall be authorized, within the limits of reasonableness, to pursue whatever action is necessary to accomplish its function.

11. The Court's decision to reserve ruling on the appointment of a master causes it to reserve ruling also on the appointment of a professional advisory committee to aid the master. Nevertheless, the Court notes that the professional mental health community in the United States has responded with enthusiasm to the pro-

eral courts are reluctant to assume control of any organization, but especially one operated by a state. This Court, always having shared that reluctance, has adhered to a policy of allowing state officials one final opportunity to perform the duties imposed upon them by law. See *e. g.*, Sims v. Amos, 336 F.Supp. 924 (M.D.Ala.1972); Nixon v. Wallace, C.A. No. 3479–N, M.D.Ala., January 22, 1972. Additionally, since the entry of the interim emergency order of March 2, 1972, defendants have worked diligently to upgrade conditions at Partlow in conformity with court-established deadlines. These factors, combined with defendants' expressed intent that the present order will be implemented forthwith and in good faith, cause the Court to withhold its decision on the appointments. Nevertheless, this Court notes, and the evidence demonstrates convincingly, that the operation of Partlow suffers from a virtual absence of administrative and managerial organization. This long-enduring organizational deficiency has been intensified by the lack of dynamic, permanent leadership. Regrettably, the problem has remained unresolved over the span of this litigation and, indeed, has been compounded by the appointment of acting and interim superintendents. The massive program of reform and reorganization to be launched at Partlow requires the guidance of a professionally qualified and experienced administrator. Consequently, this Court will order that defendants employ such an individual on a permanent basis. Should defendants

fail to do so, or otherwise fail to comply timely with the provisions of this decree, the Court will be obligated to appoint a master.

[6] The Court also reserves ruling upon plaintiffs' motion that defendant Mental Health Board be directed to sell or encumber portions of its extensive land holdings. Similarly, this Court reserves ruling on plaintiffs' motion seeking an injunction against the expenditure of state funds for nonessential functions of the state, and on other aspects of plaintiffs' requested relief designed to ameliorate the financial problems incident to the effectuation of minimum medical and constitutional standards. The Court reserves these rulings despite the fact that the primitive conditions, as well as the atmosphere of futility and despair which envelops both staff and residents at Partlow, can be attributed largely to dire shortages of operating funds. By withholding its decisions, the Court continues to observe its longstanding policy of deferring to state organizations and officials charged by law with specified responsibilities. The responsibility for appropriate funding ultimately must fall, of course, upon the State Legislature and, only to a lesser degree, upon the defendant Mental Health Board. Unfortunately, never, since the founding of Partlow in 1923, has the Legislature adequately provided for that institution.[12] The result of almost fifty years of legislative neglect has been catastrophic; atrocities occur daily.[13] Although, in fairness, the

---

posed initiation of such a committee to assist in the upgrading of Alabama's mental retardation services. Consequently, this Court strongly recommends to defendants that they develop a professional advisory committee comprised of amenable professionals from throughout the country who are able to provide the expertise the evidence reflects is important to the successful implementation of this order.

12. By defendants' admission, Partlow State School and Hospital always has been a "step-child" of the state—never having received the public support it so desperate-

ly required. Not until the short term in office of Governor Lurleen Wallace was any emphasis placed upon securing adequate care for Alabama's mentally retarded. Beginning with Mrs. Wallace's tenure in 1966, the budget for mental health has increased but remains woefully short of the minimum required for constitutional care.

13. A few of the atrocious incidents cited at the hearing in this case include the following: (a) a resident was scalded to death by hydrant water; (b) a resident was restrained in a strait jacket for nine years in order to prevent hand and finger

present State Legislature can be faulted relatively little for the crisis situation at Partlow, only that body can rectify the gross omissions of past Legislatures. To shrink from its constitutional obligation at this critical juncture would be to sanction the inhumane conditions which plague the mentally retarded of Alabama. The gravity and immediacy of the situation cannot be overemphasized. At stake is the very preservation of human life and dignity. Consequently, a prompt response from the State Legislature, as well as from the Mental Health Board and other responsible state officials, is imperative.

In the event, though, that the Legislature fails to satisfy its well-defined constitutional obligation and the Mental Health Board, because of lack of funding or any other legally insufficient reason, fails to implement fully the standards herein ordered, it will be necessary for the Court to take affirmative steps, including appointing a master, to ensure that proper funding is realized [14] and that adequate habilitation is available for the mentally retarded of Alabama.

Finally, the Court has determined that this case requires the awarding of a reasonable attorneys' fee to plaintiffs' counsel. The basis for the award and the amount thereof will be considered and treated in a separate order. The fee will be charged against the defendants as a part of the court costs in this case.

To assist the Court in its determination of how to proceed henceforth, defendants will be directed to prepare and file a report within six months from the date of this decree detailing the implementation of each standard herein

ordered. This report shall be comprehensive and shall include a statement of the progress made on each standard not yet completely implemented, specifying the reasons for incomplete performance. The report shall include also a statement of the financing secured since the issuance of this decree and of defendants' plans for procuring whatever additional financing might be required. Upon the basis of this report and other information available, the Court will evaluate defendants' work and, in due course, determine the appropriateness of appointing a master and of granting other requested relief.

Accordingly, it is the order, judgment, and decree of this Court:

1. That defendants be and they are hereby enjoined from failing to implement fully and with dispatch each of the standards set forth in Appendix A attached hereto and incorporated as a part of this decree;

2. That a human rights committee for Partlow State School and Hospital be and is hereby designated and appointed. The members thereof are listed in Appendix B attached hereto and incorporated herein. This committee shall have the purposes, functions, and spheres of operation previously set forth in this order. The members of the committee shall be paid on a per diem basis and be reimbursed for travel expenses at the same rate as members of the Alabama Board of Mental Health;

3. That defendants, within 60 days from this date, employ a professionally qualified and experienced administrator to serve Partlow State School and Hospital on a permanent basis;

---

sucking; (c) a resident was inappropriately confined in seclusion for a period of years, and (d) a resident died from the insertion by another resident of a running water hose into his rectum. Each of these incidents could have been avoided had adequate staff and facilities been available.

14. The Court realizes that the Legislature is not due back in regular session until May, 1973. Nevertheless, special ses-

sions of the Legislature are frequent occurrences in Alabama, and there has never been a time when such a session was more urgently required. If the Legislature does not act promptly to appropriate the necessary funding for mental health, the Court will be compelled to grant plaintiffs' motion to add various state officials and agencies as additional parties to this litigation and to utilize other avenues of fund raising.

4. That defendants, within six months from this date, prepare and file with this Court a report reflecting in detail the progress on the implementation of this order. This report shall be comprehensive and precise and shall explain the reasons for incomplete performance in the event the defendants have not met a standard in its entirety. The report also shall include a financial statement and an up-to-date timetable for full compliance;

5. That the court costs incurred in this proceeding, including a reasonable attorneys' fee for plaintiffs' lawyers be and they are hereby taxed against the defendants;

6. That jurisdiction of this cause be and the same is hereby specifically retained.

It is further ordered that a ruling on plaintiffs' motion for further relief, including the appointment of a master, filed March 15, 1972, be and the same is hereby reserved.

APPENDIX A

MINIMUM CONSTITUTIONAL STANDARDS FOR ADEQUATE HABILITATION OF THE MENTALLY RETARDED

I. *Definitions*

The terms used herein below are defined as follows:

a. "Institution"—Partlow State School and Hospital.

b. "Residents"—All persons who are now confined and all persons who may in the future be confined at Partlow State School and Hospital.

c. "Qualified Mental Retardation Professional"—

(1) a psychologist with a doctoral or master's degree from an accredited program and with specialized training or one year's experience in treating the mentally retarded;

(2) a physician licensed to practice in the State of Alabama, with specialized training or one's year's experience in treating the mentally retarded;

(3) an educator with a master's degree in special education from an accredited program;

(4) a social worker with a master's degree from an accredited program and with specialized training or one year's experience in working with the mentally retarded;

(5) a physical, vocational or occupational therapist licensed to practice in the State of Alabama who is a graduate of an accredited program in physical, vocational or occupational therapy, with specialized training or one year's experience in treating the mentally retarded;

(6) a registered nurse with specialized training or one year of experience treating the mentally retarded under the supervision of a Qualified Mental Retardation Professional.

d. "Resident Care Worker"—an employee of the institution, other than a Qualified Mental Retardation Professional, whose duties require regular contact with or supervision of residents.

e. "Habilitation"—the process by which the staff of the institution assists the resident to acquire and maintain those life skills which enable him to cope more effectively with the demands of his own person and of his environment and to raise the level of his physical, mental, and social efficiency. Habilitation includes but is not limited to programs of formal, structured education and treatment.

f. "Education"—the process of formal training and instruction to facilitate the intellectual and emotional development of residents.

g. "Treatment"—the prevention, amelioration and/or cure of a resident's physical disabilities or illnesses.

h. "Guardian"—a general guardian of a resident, unless the general guardian is missing, indifferent to the welfare of the resident or has an interest adverse to the resident. In such a case, *guardian* shall be defined as an individual appointed by an appropriate court on the motion of the superintendent, such guardian not to be in the control or in the employ of the Alabama Board of Mental Health.

i. "Express and Informed Consent"— the uncoerced decision of a resident who has comprehension and can signify assent or dissent.

II. *Adequate Habilitation of Residents*

1. Residents shall have a right to habilitation, including medical treatment, education and care, suited to their needs, regardless of age, degree of retardation or handicapping condition.

2. Each resident has a right to a habilitation program which will maximize his human abilities and enhance his ability to cope with his environment. The institution shall recognize that each resident, regardless of ability or status, is entitled to develop and realize his fullest potential. The institution shall implement the principle of normalization so that each resident may live as normally as possible.

3. a. No person shall be admitted to the institution unless a prior determination shall have been made [1] that residence in the institution is the least restrictive habilitation setting feasible for that person.

b. No mentally retarded person shall be admitted to the institution if services and programs in the community can afford adequate habilitation to such person.

c. Residents shall have a right to the least restrictive conditions necessary to achieve the purposes of habilitation. To this end, the institution shall make every attempt to move residents from (1) more to less structured living; (2) larger to smaller facilities; (3) larger to smaller living units; (4) group to individual residence; (5) segregated from the community to integrated into the community living; (6) dependent to independent living.

4. No borderline or mildly mentally retarded person shall be a resident of the institution. For purposes of this standard, a borderline retarded person is defined as an individual who is functioning between one and two standard deviations below the mean on a standardized intelligence test such as the Stanford Binet Scale and on measures of adaptive behavior such as the American Association on Mental Deficiency Adaptive Behavior Scale. A mildly retarded person is defined as an individual who is functioning between two and three standard deviations below the mean on a standardized intelligence test such as the Stanford Binet Scale and on a measure of adaptive behavior such as the American Association on Mental Deficiency Adaptive Behavior Scale.

5. Residents shall have a right to receive suitable educational services regardless of chronological age, degree of retardation or accompanying disabilities or handicaps.

a. The institution shall formulate a written statement of educational objectives that is consistent with the institution's mission as set forth in Standard 2, *supra*, and the other standards proposed herein.

b. School-age residents shall be provided a full and suitable educational program. Such educational program

---

1. See Standard 7, *infra.*

shall meet the following minimum standards:

	Mild [2]	Moderate	Severe/ Profound
(1) Class Size	12	9	6
(2) Length of school year (in months)	9–10	9–10	11–12
(3) Minimum length of school day (in hours)	6	6	6

6. Residents shall have a right to receive prompt and adequate medical treatment for any physical ailments and for the prevention of any illness or disability. Such medical treatment shall meet standards of medical practice in the community.

III. *Individualized Habilitation Plans*

7. Prior to his admission to the institution, each resident shall have a comprehensive social, psychological, educational, and medical diagnosis and evaluation by appropriate specialists to determine if admission is appropriate.

    a. Unless such preadmission evaluation has been conducted within three months prior to the admission, each resident shall have a new evaluation at the institution to determine if admission is appropriate.

    b. When undertaken at the institution, preadmission diagnosis and evaluation shall be completed within five days.

8. Within 14 days of his admission to the institution, each resident shall have an evaluation by appropriate specialists for programming purposes.

9. Each resident shall have an individualized habilitation plan formulated by the institution. This plan shall be developed by appropriate Qualified Mental Retardation Professionals and implemented as soon as possible but no later than 14 days after the resident's admission to the institution. An interim program of habilitation, based on the preadmission evaluation conducted pursuant to Standard 7, *supra,* shall commence promptly upon the resident's admission. Each individualized habilitation plan shall contain:

    a. a statement of the nature of the specific limitations and specific needs of the resident;

    b. a description of intermediate and long-range habilitation goals with a projected timetable for their attainment;

    c. a statement of, and an explanation for, the plan of habilitation for achieving these intermediate and long-range goals;

    d. a statement of the least restrictive setting for habilitation necessary to achieve the habilitation goals of the resident;

    e. a specification of the professionals and other staff members who are responsible for the particular resident's attaining these habilitation goals;

    f. criteria for release to less restrictive settings for habilitation, including criteria for discharge and a projected date for discharge.

10. As part of his habilitation plan, each resident shall have an individualized post-institutionalization plan. This plan shall be developed by a Qualified Mental Retardation Professional who shall begin preparation of such plan prior to the resident's admission to the institution and shall complete such plan as soon as practicable. The guardian or next of kin of the resident and the resident, if able to give informed consent, shall be consulted in the development of such plan and shall be informed of the content of such plan.

2. As is reflected in Standard 4, *supra,* it is contemplated that no mildly retarded persons be residents of the institution. However, until those mildly retarded who are presently residents are removed to more suitable locations and/or facilities, some provision must be made for their educational program.

11. In the interests of continuity of care, one Qualified Mental Retardation Professional shall be responsible for supervising the implementation of the habilitation plan, integrating the various aspects of the habilitation program, and recording the resident's progress as measured by objective indicators. This Qualified Mental Retardation Professional shall also be responsible for ensuring that the resident is released when appropriate to a less restrictive habilitation setting.

12. The habilitation plan shall be continuously reviewed by the Qualified Mental Retardation Professional responsible for supervising the implementation of the plan and shall be modified if necessary. In addition, six months after admission and at least annually thereafter, each resident shall receive a comprehensive psychological, social, educational and medical diagnosis and evaluation, and his habilitation plan shall be reviewed by an interdisciplinary team of no less than two Qualified Mental Retardation Professionals and such resident care workers as are directly involved in his habilitation and care.

13. In addition to habilitation for mental disorders, people confined at mental health institutions also are entitled to and shall receive appropriate treatment for physical illnesses such as tuberculosis.[3] In providing medical care, the State Board of Mental Health shall take advantage of whatever community-based facilities are appropriate and available and shall coordinate the resident's habilitation for mental retardation with his medical treatment.

14. Complete records for each resident shall be maintained and shall be readily available to Qualified Mental Retardation Professionals and to the resident care workers who are directly involved with the particular resident. All information contained in a resident's records shall be considered privileged and confidential. The guardian, next of kin, and any person properly authorized in writing by the resident, if such resident is capable of giving informed consent, or by his guardian or next of kin, shall be permitted access to the resident's records. These records shall include:

a. Identification data, including the resident's legal status;

b. The resident's history, including but not limited to:

(1) family data, educational background, and employment record;

(2) prior medical history, both physical and mental, including prior institutionalization;

c. The resident's grievances if any;

d. An inventory of the resident's life skills;

e. A record of each physical examination which describes the results of the examination;

f. A copy of the individual habilitation plan and any modifications thereto and an appropriate summary which will guide and assist the resident care workers in implementing the resident's program;

g. The findings made in periodic reviews of the habilitation plan (see Standard 12, *supra*), which findings shall include an analysis of the successes and failures of the habilitation program and shall direct whatever modifications are necessary;

h. A copy of the post-institutionalization plan and any modifications thereto, and a summary of the steps that have been taken to implement that plan;

i. A medication history and status, pursuant to Standard 22, *infra*;

---

3. Approximately 50 patients at Bryce-Searcy are tubercular as also are approximately four residents at Partlow.

j. A summary of each significant contact by a Qualified Mental Retardation Professional with the resident;

k. A summary of the resident's response to his program, prepared by a Qualified Mental Retardation Professional involved in the resident's habilitation and recorded at least monthly. Such response, wherever possible, shall be scientifically documented.

l. A monthly summary of the extent and nature of the resident's work activities described in the Standard 33(b), *infra* and the effect of such activity upon the resident's progress along the habilitation plan;

m. A signed order by a Qualified Mental Retardation Professional for any physical restraints, as provided in Standard 26(a) (1), *infra;*

n. A description of any extraordinary incident or accident in the institution involving the resident, to be entered by a staff member noting personal knowledge of the incident or accident or other source of information, including any reports of investigations of resident mistreatment, as required by Standard 28, *infra;*

o. A summary of family visits and contacts;

p. A summary of attendance and leaves from the institution;

q. A record of any seizures, illnesses, treatments thereof, and immunizations.

IV. *Humane Physical and Psychological Environment*

15. Residents shall have a right to dignity, privacy and humane care.

16. Residents shall lose none of the rights enjoyed by citizens of Alabama and of the United States solely by reason of their admission or commitment to the institution, except as expressly determined by an appropriate court.

17. No person shall be presumed mentally incompetent solely by reason of his admission or commitment to the institution.

18. The opportunity for religious worship shall be accorded to each resident who desires such worship. Provisions for religious worship shall be made available to all residents on a nondiscriminatory basis. No individual shall be coerced into engaging in any religious activities.

19. Residents shall have the same rights to telephone communication as patients at Alabama public hospitals, except to the extent that a Qualified Mental Retardation Professional responsible for formulation of a particular resident's habilitation plan (see Standard 9, *supra*) writes an order imposing special restrictions and explains the reasons for any such restrictions. The written order must be renewed semiannually if any restrictions are to be continued. Residents shall have an unrestricted right to visitation, except to the extent that a Qualified Mental Retardation Professional responsible for formulation of a particular resident's habilitation plan (see Standard 9, *supra*) writes an order imposing special restrictions and explains the reasons for any such restrictions. The written order must be renewed semiannually if any restrictions are to be continued.

20. Residents shall be entitled to send and receive sealed mail. Moreover, it shall be the duty of the institution to facilitate the exercise of this right by furnishing the necessary materials and assistance.

21. The institution shall provide, under appropriate supervision, suitable opportunities for the resident's interaction with members of the opposite sex, except where a Qualified Mental Retardation Professional responsible for the formulation of a particular resident's habilitation plan writes an order to the contrary and explains the reasons therefor.

22. *Medication*:
    a. No medication shall be administered unless at the written order of a physician.
    b. Notation of each individual's medication shall be kept in his medical records (Standard 14(i) *supra*). At least weekly the attending physician shall review the drug regimen of each resident under his care. All prescriptions shall be written with a termination date, which shall not exceed 30 days.
    c. Residents shall have a right to be free from unnecessary or excessive medication. The resident's records shall state the effects of psychoactive medication on the resident. When dosages of such are changed or other psychoactive medications are prescribed, a notation shall be made in the resident's record concerning the effect of the new medication or new dosages and the behavior changes, if any, which occur.
    d. Medication shall not be used as punishment, for the convenience of staff, as a substitute for a habilitation program, or in quantities that interfere with the resident's habilitation program.
    e. Pharmacy services at the institution shall be directed by a professionally competent pharmacist licensed to practice in the State of Alabama. Such pharmacist shall be a graduate of a school of pharmacy accredited by the American Council on Pharmaceutical Education. Appropriate officials of the institution, at their option, may hire such a pharmacist or pharmacists fulltime or, in lieu thereof, contract with outside pharmacists.
    f. Whether employed fulltime or on a contract basis, the pharmacist shall perform duties which include but are not limited to the following:

       (1) Receiving the original, or direct copy, of the physician's drug treatment order;

       (2) Reviewing the drug regimen, and any changes, for potentially adverse reactions, allergies, interactions, contraindications, rationality, and laboratory test modifications and advising the physician of any recommended changes, with reasons and with an alternate drug regimen;

       (3) Maintaining for each resident an individual record of all medications (prescription and nonprescription) dispensed, including quantities and frequency of refills;

       (4) Participating, as appropriate, in the continuing interdisciplinary evaluation of individual residents for the purposes of initiation, monitoring, and follow-up of individualized habilitation programs.

    g. Only appropriately trained staff shall be allowed to administer drugs.

23. Seclusion, defined as the placement of a resident alone in a locked room, shall not be employed. Legitimate "time out" procedures may be utilized under close and direct professional supervision as a technique in behavior-shaping programs.

24. Behavior modification programs involving the use of noxious or aversive stimuli shall be reviewed and approved by the institution's Human Rights Committee and shall be conducted only with the express and informed consent of the affected resident, if the resident is able to give such consent, and of his guardian or next of kin, after opportunities for consultation with independent specialists and with legal counsel. Such behavior modification programs shall be conducted only under the supervision of and in the presence of a Qualified Mental Retardation Professional who has had proper training in such techniques.

25. Electric shock devices shall be considered a research technique for the purpose of these standards. Such

devices shall only be used in extraordinary circumstances to prevent self-mutilation leading to repeated and possibly permanent physical damage to the resident and only after alternative techniques have failed. The use of such devices shall be subject to the conditions prescribed in Standard 24, *supra,* and Standard 29, *infra,* and shall be used only under the direct and specific order of the superintendent.

26. Physical restraint shall be employed only when absolutely necessary to protect the resident from injury to himself or to prevent injury to others. Restraint shall not be employed as punishment, for the convenience of staff, or as a substitute for a habilitation program. Restraint shall be applied only if alternative techniques have failed and only if such restraint imposes the least possible restriction consistent with its purpose.

a. Only Qualified Mental Retardation Professionals may authorize the use of restraints.

(1) Orders for restraints by the Qualified Mental Retardation Professionals shall be in writing and shall not be in force for longer than 12 hours.

(2) A resident placed in restraint shall be checked at least every 30 minutes by staff trained in the use of restraints, and a record of such checks shall be kept.

(3) Mechanical restraints shall be designed and used so as not to cause physical injury to the resident and so as to cause the least possible discomfort.

(4) Opportunity for motion and exercise shall be provided for a period of not less than ten minutes during each two hours in which restraint is employed.

(5) Daily reports shall be made to the superintendent by those Qualified Mental Retardation Professionals ordering the use of restraints, summarizing all such uses of restraint, the types used, the duration, and the reasons therefor.

b. The institution shall cause a written statement of this policy to be posted in each living unit and circulated to all staff members.

27. Corporal punishment shall not be permitted.

28. The institution shall prohibit mistreatment, neglect or abuse in any form of any resident.

a. Alleged violations shall be reported immediately to the superintendent and there shall be a written record that:

(1) Each alleged violation has been thoroughly investigated and findings stated;

(2) The results of such investigation are reported to the superintendent and to the commissioner within 24 hours of the report of the incident. Such reports shall also be made to the institution's Human Rights Committee monthly and to the Alabama Board of Mental Health at its next scheduled public meeting.

b. The institution shall cause a written statement of this policy to be posted in each cottage and building and circulated to all staff members.

29. Residents shall have a right not to be subjected to experimental research without the express and informed consent of the resident, if the resident is able to give such consent, and of his guardian or next of kin, after opportunities for consultation with independent specialists and with legal counsel. Such proposed research shall first have been reviewed and approved by the institution's Human Rights Committee before such consent shall be sought. Prior to such approval the institution's Human Rights Committee shall determine that such research complies with the princi-

ples of the Statement on the Use of Human Subjects for Research of the American Association on Mental Deficiency and with the principles for research involving human subjects required by the United States Department of Health, Education and Welfare for projects supported by that agency.

30. Residents shall have a right not to be subjected to any unusual or hazardous treatment procedures without the express and informed consent of the resident, if the resident is able to give such consent, and of his guardian or next of kin, after opportunities for consultation with independent specialists and legal counsel. Such proposed procedures shall first have been reviewed and approved by the institution's Human Rights Committee before such consent shall be sought.

31. Residents shall have a right to regular physical exercise several times a week. It shall be the duty of the institution to provide both indoor and outdoor facilities and equipment for such exercise.

32. Residents shall have a right to be outdoors daily in the absence of contrary medical considerations.

33. The following rules shall govern resident labor:

a. *Institution Maintenance*

(1) No resident shall be required to perform labor which involves the operation and maintenance of the institution or for which the institution is under contract with an outside organization. Privileges or release from the institution shall not be conditioned upon the performance of labor covered by this provision. Residents may voluntarily engage in such labor if the labor is compensated in accordance with the minimum wage laws of the Fair Labor Standards Act, 29 U.S.C. § 206 as amended, 1966.

(2) No resident shall be involved in the care (feeding, clothing, bath-

ing), training, or supervision of other residents unless he:

(a) has volunteered;

(b) has been specifically trained in the necessary skills;

(c) has the humane judgment required for such activities;

(d) is adequately supervised; and

(e) is reimbursed in accordance with the minimum wage laws of the Fair Labor Standards Act, 29 U.S.C. § 206 as amended, 1966.

b. *Training Tasks and Labor*

(1) Residents may be required to perform vocational training tasks which do not involve the operation and maintenance of the institution, subject to a presumption that an assignment of longer than three months to any task is not a training task, provided the specific task or any change in task assignment is:

(a) An integrated part of the resident's habilitation plan and approved as a habilitation activity by a Qualified Mental Retardation Professional responsible for supervising the resident's habilitation;

(b) Supervised by a staff member to oversee the habilitation aspects of the activity.

(2) Residents may voluntarily engage in habilitative labor at non-program hours for which the institution would otherwise have to pay an employee, provided the specific labor or any change in labor is:

(a) An integrated part of the resident's habilitation plan and approved as a habilitation activity by a Qualified Mental Retardation Professional responsible for supervising the resident's habilitation;

(b) Supervised by a staff member to oversee the habilitation aspects of the activity; and

(c) Compensated in accordance with the minimum wage laws of the Fair Labor Standards Act, 29 U.S.C. § 206 as amended, 1966.

c. *Personal Housekeeping* Residents may be required to perform tasks of a personal housekeeping nature such as the making of one's own bed.

d. Payment to residents pursuant to this paragraph shall not be applied to the costs of institutionalization.

e. Staffing shall be sufficient so that the institution is not dependent upon the use of residents or volunteers for the care, maintenance or habilitation of other residents or for income-producing services. The institution shall formulate a written policy to protect the residents from exploitation when they are engaged in productive work.

34. A nourishing, well-balanced diet shall be provided each resident.

a. The diet for residents shall provide at a minimum the Recommended Daily Dietary Allowance as developed by the National Academy of Sciences. Menus shall be satisfying and shall provide the Recommended Daily Dietary Allowances. In developing such menus, the institution shall utilize the Moderate Cost Food Plan of the United States Department of Agriculture. The institution shall not spend less per patient for raw food, including the value of donated food, than the most recent per person costs of the Moderate Cost Food Plan for the Southern Region of the United States, as compiled by the United States Department of Agriculture, for appropriate groupings of residents, discounted for any savings which might result from institutional procurement of such food.

b. Provision shall be made for special therapeutic diets and for substitutes at the request of the resident, or his guardian or next of kin, in accordance with the religious requirements of any resident's faith.

c. Denial of a nutritionally adequate diet shall not be used as punishment.

d. Residents, except for the non-mobile, shall eat or be fed in dining rooms.

35. Each resident shall have an adequate allowance of neat, clean, suitably fitting and seasonable clothing.

a. Each resident shall have his own clothing, which is properly and inconspicuously marked with his name, and he shall be kept dressed in this clothing. The institution has an obligation to supply an adequate allowance of clothing to any residents who do not have suitable clothing of their own. Residents shall have the opportunity to select from various types of neat, clean, and seasonable clothing. Such clothing shall be considered the resident's throughout his stay in the institution.

b. Clothing both in amount and type shall make it possible for residents to go out of doors in inclement weather, to go for trips or visits appropriately dressed, and to make a normal appearance in the community.

c. Nonambulatory residents shall be dressed daily in their own clothing, including shoes, unless contraindicated in written medical orders.

d. Washable clothing shall be designed for multiply handicapped residents being trained in self-help skills, in accordance with individual needs.

e. Clothing for incontinent residents shall be designed to foster comfortable sitting, crawling and/or walking, and toilet training.

f. A current inventory shall be kept of each resident's personal and clothing items.

g. The institution shall make provision for the adequate and regular laundering of the residents' clothing.

36. Each resident shall have the right to keep and use his own personal possessions except insofar as such clothes or personal possessions may be determined to be dangerous, either to himself or to others, by a Qualified Mental Retardation Professional.

37. a. Each resident shall be assisted in learning normal grooming practices

with individual toilet articles, including soap and toothpaste, that are available to each resident.

b. Teeth shall be brushed daily with an effective dentifrice. Individual brushes shall be properly marked, used, and stored.

c. Each resident shall have a shower or tub bath, at least daily, unless medically contraindicated.

d. Residents shall be regularly scheduled for hair cutting and styling, in an individualized manner, by trained personnel.

e. For residents who require such assistance, cutting of toe nails and fingernails shall be scheduled at regular intervals.

38. *Physical Facilities* A resident has a right to a humane physical environment within the institutional facilities. These facilities shall be designed to make a positive contribution to the efficient attainment of the habilitation goals of the institution.

a. *Resident Unit* All ambulatory residents shall sleep in single rooms or in multi-resident rooms of no more than six persons. The number of nonambulatory residents in a multi-resident room shall not exceed ten persons. There shall be allocated a minimum of 80 square feet of floor space per resident in a multi-resident room. Screens or curtains shall be provided to ensure privacy. Single rooms shall have a minimum of 100 square feet of floor space. Each resident shall be furnished with a comfortable bed with adequate changes of linen, a closet or locker for his personal belongings, and appropriate furniture such as a chair and a bedside table, unless contraindicated by a Qualified Mental Retardation Professional who shall state the reasons for any such restriction.

b. *Toilets and Lavatories* There shall be one toilet and one lavatory for each six residents. A lavatory shall be provided with each toilet facility. The toilets shall be installed in separate stalls for ambulatory residents, or in curtained areas for non-ambulatory residents, to ensure privacy, shall be clean and free of odor, and shall be equipped with appropriate safety devices for the physically handicapped. Soap and towels and/or drying mechanisms shall be available in each lavatory. Toilet paper shall be available in each toilet facility.

c. *Showers* There shall be one tub or shower for each eight residents. If a central bathing area is provided, each tub or shower shall be divided by curtains to ensure privacy. Showers and tubs shall be equipped with adequate safety accessories.

d. *Day Room* The minimum day room area shall be 40 square feet per resident. Day rooms shall be attractive and adequately furnished with reading lamps, tables, chairs, television, radio and other recreational facilities. They shall be conveniently located to residents' bedrooms and shall have outside windows. There shall be at least one day room area on each bedroom floor in a multi-story facility. Areas used for corridor traffic shall not be counted as day room space; nor shall a chapel with fixed pews be counted as a day room area.

e. *Dining Facilities* The minimum dining room area shall be ten square feet per resident. The dining room shall be separate from the kitchen and shall be furnished with comfortable chairs and tables with hard, washable surfaces.

157

f. *Linen Servicing and Handling* The institution shall provide adequate facilities and equipment for the expeditious handling of clean and soiled bedding and other linen. There must be frequent changes of bedding and other linen, but in any event no less than every seven days, to assure sanitation and resident comfort. After soiling by an incontinent resident, bedding and linen must be immediately changed and removed from the living unit. Soiled linen and laundry shall be removed from the living unit daily.

g. *Housekeeping* Regular housekeeping and maintenance procedures which will ensure that the institution is maintained in a safe, clean, and attractive condition shall be developed and implemented.

h. *Nonambulatory Residents* There must be special facilities for nonambulatory residents to assure their safety and comfort, including special fittings on toilets and wheelchairs. Appropriate provision shall be made to permit nonambulatory residents to communicate their needs to staff.

i. *Physical Plant*

(1) Pursuant to an established routine maintenance and repair program, the physical plant shall be kept in a continuous state of good repair and operation so as to ensure the health, comfort, safety and well-being of the residents and so as not to impede in any manner the habilitation programs of the residents.

(2) Adequate heating, air conditioning and ventilation systems and equipment shall be afforded to maintain temperatures and air changes which are required for the comfort of residents at all times. Ventilation systems shall be adequate to remove steam and offensive odors or to mask such odors. The temperature in the institution shall not exceed 83°F nor fall below 68°F.

(3) Thermostatically controlled hot water shall be provided in adequate quantities and maintained at the required temperature for resident use (110°F at the fixture) and for mechanical dishwashing and laundry use (180°F at the equipment). Thermostatically controlled hot water valves shall be equipped with a double valve system that provides both auditory and visual signals of valve failures.

(4) Adequate refuse facilities shall be provided so that solid waste, rubbish and other refuse will be collected and disposed of in a manner which will prohibit transmission of disease and not create a nuisance or fire hazard or provide a breeding place for rodents and insects.

(5) The physical facilities must meet all fire and safety standards established by the state and locality. In addition, the institution shall meet such provisions of the Life Safety Code of the National Fire Protection Association (21st edition, 1967) as are applicable to it.

V. *Qualified Staff in Numbers Sufficient to Provide Adequate Habilitation*

39. Each Qualified Mental Retardation Professional and each physician shall meet all licensing and certification requirements promulgated by the State of Alabama for persons engaged in private practice of the same profession elsewhere in Alabama. Other staff members shall meet the same licensing and certification requirements as persons who engage in private practice of their specialty elsewhere in Alabama.

a. All resident care workers who have not had prior clinical experience in a mental retardation institution shall have suitable orientation training.

b. Staff members on all levels shall have suitable, regularly scheduled in-service training.

40. Each resident care worker shall be under the direct professional supervision of a Qualified Mental Retardation Professional.

41. *Staffing Ratios*

a. Qualified staff in numbers sufficient to administer adequate habilitation shall be provided. Such staffing shall include but not be limited to the following fulltime professional and special services. Qualified Mental Retardation Professionals trained in particular disciplines may in appropriate situations perform services or functions traditionally performed by members of other disciplines. Substantial changes in staff deployment may be made with the prior approval of this Court upon a clear and convincing demonstration that the proposed deviation from this staffing structure would enhance the habilitation of the residents. Professional staff shall possess the qualifications of Qualified Mental Retardation Professionals as defined herein unless expressly stated otherwise.

			Severe/
b. *Unit*	Mild [4]	Moderate	Profound
	60	60	60
(1) Psychologists	1:60	1:60	1:60
(2) Social Workers	1:60	1:60	1:60
(3) Special Educators (shall include an equal number of master's degree and bachelor's degree holders in special education)	1:15	1:10	1:30
(4) Vocational Therapists	1:60	1:60	—

	Mild	Moderate	Severe/Profound
(5) Recreational Therapists (shall be master's degree graduates from an accredited program)	1:60	1:60	1:60
(6) Occupational Therapists	—	—	1:60
(7) Registered Nurses	1:60	1:60	1:12
(8) Resident Care Workers	1:2.5	1:1.25	1:1

The following professional staff shall be fulltime employees of the institution who shall not be assigned to a single unit but who shall be available to meet the needs of any resident of the institution:

Physicians	1:200
Physical Therapists	1:100
Speech & Hearing Therapists	1:100
Dentists [5]	1:200
Social Workers (shall be principally involved in the placement of residents in the community and shall include bachelor's degree graduates from an accredited program in social work)	1:80
Chaplains [6]	1:200

c. Qualified medical specialists of recognized professional ability shall be available for specialized care and consultation. Such specialist services shall include a psychiatrist on a one-day per week basis, a physiatrist on a two-day per week basis, and any other medical or health-related specialty available in the community.

VI. *Miscellaneous*

42. The guardian or next of kin of each resident shall promptly, upon resident's admission, receive a written copy of all the above standards for adequate habilitation. Each resident, if the resident is able to comprehend, shall promptly upon his admission be orally informed in clear language of the above standards and, where appropriate, be provided with a written copy.

43. The superintendent shall report in writing to the next of kin or guardian of the resident at least every six months on the resident's educational, vocational and living skills progress and medical condition. Such report shall also state any appropriate habilitation program which has

4. See n. 2, *supra.*

5. Defendants may, in lieu of employing fulltime dentists, contract outside the institution for dental care. In this event the dental services provided the residents must include (a) complete dental examinations and appropriate corrective dental work for

each resident each six months and (b) a dentist on call 24 hours per day for emergency work.

6. Defendants may, in lieu of employing fulltime chaplains, recruit, upon the ratio shown above, interfaith volunteer chaplains.

not been afforded to the resident because of inadequate habilitation resources.

44. a. No resident shall be subjected to a behavior modification program designed to eliminate a particular pattern of behavior without prior certification by a physician that he has examined the resident in regard to behavior to be extinguished and finds that such behavior is not caused by a physical condition which could be corrected by appropriate medical procedures.

b. No resident shall be subjected to a behavior modification program which attempts to extinguish socially appropriate behavior or to develop new behavior patterns when such behavior modifications serve only institutional convenience.

45. No resident shall have any of his organs removed for the purpose of transplantation without compliance with the procedures set forth in Standard 30, *supra,* and after a court hearing on such transplantation in which the resident is represented by a guardian *ad litem.* This standard shall apply to any other surgical procedure which is undertaken for reasons other than therapeutic benefit to the resident.

46. Within 90 days of the date of this order, each resident of the institution shall be evaluated as to his mental, emotional, social, and physical condition. Such evaluation or reevaluation shall be conducted by an interdisciplinary team of Qualified Mental Retardation Professionals who shall use professionally recognized tests and examination procedures. Each resident's guardian, next of kin or legal representative shall be contacted and his readiness to make provisions for the resident's care in the community shall be ascertained. Each resident shall be returned to his family, if adequately habilitated, or assigned to the least restrictive habilitation setting.

47. Each resident discharged to the community shall have a program of transitional habilitation assistance.

48. The institution shall continue to suspend any new admissions of residents until all of the above standards of adequate habilitation have been met.

49. No person shall be admitted to any publicly supported residential institution caring for mentally retarded persons unless such institution meets the above standards.

APPENDIX B
PARTLOW HUMAN RIGHTS COMMITTEE

1. Ms. Harriet S. Tillman—Chairman —3544 Brookwood Road, Birmingham, Alabama

2. Dr. J. W. Benton —3008 Brook Hollow Lane, Birmingham, Alabama

3. Mr. Paul R. Davis —Tuscaloosa News, Tuscaloosa, Alabama 35401

4. Reverend Robert Keever —University Presbyterian Church, Tuscaloosa, Alabama 35401

5. Ms. Nancy Poole —1836 Dorchester, Birmingham, Alabama

6. Mr. Eugene Ward —c/o Partlow State School and Hospital, Tuscaloosa, Alabama 35401

7. Ms. Estelle Witherspoon —Alberta, Alabama 36720

IN THE UNITED STATES DISTRICT COURT FOR THE MIDDLE
DISTRICT OF ALABAMA, NORTHERN DIVISION

Ricky WYATT, by and through
his aunt and legal guardian,
Mrs. W. C. Rawlins, Jr., et al.,
for themselves jointly and severally and for all others similarly situated,

Plaintiffs,

v.

Dr. Stonewall B. STICKNEY,
as Commissioner of Mental
Health and the State of Alabama Mental Health Officer,
et al.

Defendants,
United States of America et al.,
Amici Curiae.

CIVIL ACTION NO. 3195–N

———◆———

On Request for Attorneys' Fees

[7] Once again this Court is confronted with a request for attorneys'
fees made by plaintiffs involved in *pro
bono publico* litigation, and the request
is well taken.[1] In 1967, over three years
prior to the initiation of this suit, the
American Association on Mental Deficiency [hereinafter referred to as
AAMD] conducted a study of Partlow
State School and Hospital.[2] That study,
which was made available to Partlow's
Director and to the State Mental Health
Board, portrayed the institution as one
enveloped by an atmosphere of despair,
hopelessness and depression. The AAMD
found Partlow grossly deficient virtually
in every respect, including habilitation
programming, staffing, staff training,
community relations and residential facilities. At the time of the study, Partlow's administration and organization
were found to be chaotic. The institution had promulgated no statement of
its philosophy and objectives, and what

emergency and safety procedures existed
were evaluated as primitive and ineffective. Evidence offered at trial demonstrated that defendants also had knowledge prior to the initiation of this suit
of the unconstitutionally substandard
conditions at Bryce and Searcy Hospitals.
Nevertheless, although many of the inadequacies known by defendants to exist
in Alabama's mental health institutions
could have been corrected without large
expenditures, little, if any, progress toward upgrading conditions was realized
until this case was initiated. From a
legal standpoint, such nonfeasance on the
part of defendants constitutes bad faith
which necessitated the expense of litigation. This bad faith forms a valid basis
for the granting of attorneys' fees. See
e. g., Vaughan v. Atkinson, 369 U.S. 527,
530–531, 82 S.Ct. 997, 8 L.Ed.2d 88
(1961).

[8] A second, and more appropriate,
justification for the Court's award, however, evolves from a kind of benefit

1. Other such cases in which this Court has
found a valid basis for the awarding of a
reasonable attorneys' fee include Sims v.
Amos, 336 F.Supp. 924 (M.D.Ala.1972)
(three judges) and NAACP v. Allen, 340
F.Supp. 703 (M.D.Ala.1972).

2. American Ass'n on Mental Deficiency Institutional Evaluation Project, Final Report For Partlow State School & Hospital
(1967).

theory. See Mills v. Electro Auto-Lite Co., 396 U.S. 375, 90 S.Ct. 616, 24 L.Ed. 2d 593 (1970). Plaintiffs bringing suits to enforce a strong national policy often benefit a class of people far broader than those actually involved in the litigation. Such plaintiffs, who are said to act as "private attorneys general," Newman v. Piggie Park Enterprises, Inc., 390 U.S. 400, 88 S.Ct. 964, 19 L.Ed.2d 1263 (1968), rarely recover significant damage awards. Moreover, if a violation of civil rights is alleged or if some other challenge to constituted authority is involved, these plaintiffs and their attorneys may confront other, more personal obstacles to the maintenance of their public-minded suits. See NAACP v. Allen, 340 F.Supp. 703 (M.D.Ala.1972). Consequently, in order to eliminate the impediments to *pro bono publico* litigation and to carry out congressional policy, an award of attorneys' fees not only is essential but also is legally required. See Lee v. Southern Home Sites, 444 F.2d 143 (5th Cir. 1971); Sims v. Amos, 336 F.Supp. 924 (M.D.Ala.1972); NAACP v. Allen, supra; Bradley v. School Bd. of Richmond, 53 F.R.D. 28 (E.D.Va.1971).

The present action clearly is one intended to be encouraged by the benefit rule. By successfully prosecuting this suit, plaintiffs have benefitted not only the present residents of Bryce, Partlow and Searcy but also everyone who will be confined to those institutions in the future. Veritably, it is no overstatement to assert that all of Alabama's citizens have profited and will continue to profit from this litigation. So prevalent are mental disorders in our society that no family is immune from their perilous incursion. Consequently, the availability of institutions capable of dealing successfully with such disorders is essential and, of course, in the best interest of all Alabamians.

[9] Despite plaintiffs' having benefitted so many people, however, they neither sought nor recovered any damages. Nevertheless, the expenses they incurred in vindicating the public good were considerable. To burden only plaintiffs with these costs not only is unfair but also is legally impermissible. See e. g., Mills v. Electro Auto-Lite Co., supra; Lee v. Southern Home Sites, supra. Considerations of equity require that those who profit share the expense. In this case, the most logical way to spread the burden among those benefitted is to grant attorneys' fees. Plaintiffs clearly are entitled to a reasonable award.

[10, 11] This Court must consider, therefore, what is reasonable under the circumstances. Factors relevant to the Court's determination generally are the same as those covering grants of attorneys' fees in commercial cases. See Bradley v. School Bd. of Richmond, supra. They include the intricacy of the case and the difficulty of proof, the time reasonably expended in the preparation and trial of the case, the degree of competence displayed by the attorneys seeking compensation and the measure of success achieved by these attorneys. In public interest cases, courts also should consider the benefit inuring to the public, the personal hardships that bringing this kind of litigation causes plaintiffs and their lawyers, and the added responsibility of representing a class rather than only individual plaintiffs.

Having considered these factors, the Court notes that the several aspects of the present litigation have synthesized to compose a very complex case. Plaintiffs' attorneys have navigated through a heretofore uncharted course and, in the process, have helped establish minimum constitutional standards for mental health institutions. These attorneys have exhibited professional conscientiousness throughout the litigation, and their toil, along with that of others, has culminated in an incalculable benefit to the people of Alabama.[3]

3. The able and invaluable assistance which plaintiffs' attorneys received from amici in this case in no way detracts from the quality of their effort. The Court is con-

strained, however, to comment generally on the number of lawyers for whom plaintiffs seek attorneys' fees. Because this case is so complex and the time required

The above considerations, and others, militate in favor of the Court's granting plaintiffs' attorneys full compensation. Nevertheless, the weight of these factors must be balanced against and tempered by the nature of this lawsuit. It is the duty of members of the legal profession to represent clients who are unable to pay for counsel and also to bring suits in the public interest. While lawyers who satisfy this ethical responsibility should be remunerated, their fees should not be exorbitant. This Court must bear in mind that the very goals plaintiffs' attorneys seek to achieve through litigation require great monetary outlays, most of which presently are unavailable. Some compromise, therefore, is essential.

In attempting to determine what is a reasonable fee under the circumstances, this Court is impressed with the philosophy underlying the Criminal Justice Act. That Act provides for compensation to attorneys appointed to represent indigent criminal defendants. The Act's legislative history makes clear that although the amount provided, $30 per in-court hour and $20 per out-of-court hour, is below normal levels of compensation in legal practice, it nevertheless is considered a reasonable basis upon which lawyers can carry out their professional responsibility without either personal profiteering or undue financial sacrifice. 1964 U.S.Code Cong. & Admin. News, p. 2997.

The Court is convinced that this philosophy applies with equal force to the present case. As already emphasized, lawyers participating in the case *sub judice*, as well as those participating in a Criminal Justice Act case, perform ethical and professional responsibilities. In both cases they embark upon their participation with knowledge that their named clients are unable to pay them. Generally, however, these lawyers are not motivated by desire for profit but by public spirit and sense of duty. Moreover, in both cases the rights involved, those dealing with restrictions on physical freedom, are of the most profound significance to the public. These similarities justify referral to the Criminal Justice Act.

[12]   On the basis of the fee schedule set forth in the Act, therefore, this Court has determined that a reasonable fee in this case is $30 per in-court hour and $20 per out-of-court hour.[4] In establishing this fee, however, the Court is careful to note that the Criminal Justice Act furnishes only a very flexible standard. In a particular case, a reasonable fee may vary either way from that provided by the Act.

In addition to determining an hourly fee, the Court is obliged to decide what time is reasonable for an attorney or attorneys to have spent in connection with the lawsuit. Plaintiffs' lawyers, Jack Drake and Reber Boult, have filed statements setting forth in detail their time expended in preparation of the case. The hours they have claimed are reasonable and uncontested. Plaintiffs' other lawyer, George Dean, however, has neglected to file a similar statement. Instead, he has testified only that he has spent almost all of 18 months working on the case. Under such circumstances, the Court must decide the amount of time an attorney should reasonably have spent to accomplish the work produced. From the evidence adduced at the hearing on this matter, the Court has made that determination.

Accordingly, it is the order, judgment and decree of this Court:

1.   That attorney's fees and expenses of the Honorable George Dean in the amount of $23,600.00 be and the same

---

to meet various deadlines so great, the Court feels that the number of lawyers utilized by plaintiffs was necessary. In another case in which attorneys' fees are appropriate, the same may not be true. The Court must decide on an ad hoc basis whether the number of attorneys employ-

ed and the time expended by them were reasonable.

4.   In addition to regularly employed legal staff, defendants retained special counsel in this case at a rate of $30 per hour.

are hereby taxed against defendant Alabama Mental Health Board;

2. That attorney's fees and expenses of the Honorable Jack Drake in the amount of $7,595.91 be and the same are hereby taxed against defendant Alabama Mental Health Board; and

3. That attorney's fees and expenses of the Honorable Reber Boult in the amount of $5,558.71 be and the same are hereby taxed against defendant Alabama Mental Health Board.

It is further ordered that defendant Alabama Mental Health Board pay said expenses and attorneys' fees to the Clerk of this Court within 30 days from this date. Upon receipt of these funds, the Clerk of this Court will deposit them in an interest bearing account. The Clerk of this Court is ordered and directed to hold said funds in said interest bearing account pending further order of this Court.

Wyatt v. Aderholt

Ricky WYATT, By and Through his aunt
and legal guardian Mrs. W. C. Rawlins,
Jr., et al., etc., Plaintiffs-Appellees,
v.
Charles ADERHOLT, as Commissioner of
Mental Health, et al., Defendants,
The Alabama Mental Health Board, an
Agency of the State of Alabama, and
George C. Wallace, as Governor of Ala.,
Defendants-Appellants.

No. 72–2634.

United States Court of Appeals,
Fifth Circuit.

Nov. 8, 1974.

WISDOM, Circuit Judge:

In this case, we must decide whether
federal district courts have the power to
order state mental institutions to provide minimum levels of psychiatric care
and treatment [1] to persons civilly committed to the institutions.

The guardians of patients civilly committed to three Alabama facilities for
the mentally handicapped brought this
class action on behalf of their wards and
other civilly committed patients at those
institutions. The Honorable Frank M.
Johnson, trial judge, held that mentally
ill patients "have a constitutional right
to receive such individual treatment as
will give each of them a reasonable opportunity to be cured or to improve his
or her mental condition". Wyatt v.
Stickney, M.D.Ala.1971, 325 F.Supp.
781, 784. In a later order, Judge Johnson held that the mentally retarded pa-

[1]. "Treatment" means care provided by mental health professionals and others that is
adequate and appropriate for the needs of the
mentally impaired inmate. Treatment also
encompasses a humane physical and psychological environment. The term "habilitation", used by the parties and amici in the
district court and by the district court in its
order of April 13, 1972 (Partlow State
School and Hospital) is a term used to de-
scribe that treatment which is appropriate

to the condition of the mental retardate.
For convenience, in this opinion we group
"habilitation" and "treatment" under the
single term "treatment", and to include
those instances where rehabilitation is impossible in which event the requirement is
minimally adequate habilitation and care, beyond the subsistence level custodial care that
would be provided in a penitentiary. Donaldson v. O'Connor, 5 Cir., 1974, 493 F.2d
507, 522.

tients have a constitutional right to "such individual habilitation as will give each of them a realistic opportunity to lead a more useful and meaningful life and to return to society". Wyatt v. Stickney, M.D.Ala.1972, 344 F.Supp. 387, 390. The district court found that conditions at the three facilities deprived the plaintiffs of these constitutional rights, and ordered the defendants-appellants, Alabama officials responsible for the administration of the state's mental health programs, to implement a detailed set of standards designed to ensure the provision of minimally adequate treatment and habilitation at the institutions. From this order, the Alabama Mental Health Board and Alabama's Governor George C. Wallace bring separate appeals.

Together, the Mental Health Board and the Governor advance six major contentions on appeal. They contend (1) that the district court erred in holding that civilly committed mental patients have a constitutional right to treatment; (2) that the court lacked jurisdiction because the suit was in effect a suit against the state proscribed by the eleventh amendment; (3) that the case involves rights and duties not susceptible to determination by judicially ascertainable and manageable standards, and therefore presents a non-justiciable controversy; (4) that the order of the district court invades a province of decision-making exclusively reserved to the state legislature; (5) that the plaintiffs were not entitled to equitable relief because they had adequate remedies at law to protect the rights they asserted; and (6) that the district court erred in awarding plaintiffs a reasonable attorneys' fee.

Neither in the district court nor on appeal to this Court have the defendants challenged the detailed set of standards articulated by the district court. They have conceded that if there is a constitu-

tional right to treatment enforceable by a suit for injunctive relief in federal court, those standards accurately reflect what would be required to ensure the provision of adequate treatment.

I.

A. *The proceedings below*

This case began innocuously enough, when a cut in the Alabama cigarette tax forced the state to fire 99 professional, subprofessional, and intern employees [2] at the Bryce Hospital, a state-run institution for the mentally ill at Tuscaloosa. The plaintiffs filed their complaint October 23, 1970. The complaint named two classes as plaintiffs. One, represented by Ricky Wyatt and two other named plaintiffs, appellees here, consisted of the patients at Bryce. The other, represented by five of the then recently terminated employees, consisted of the employees who had been dismissed for budgetary reasons. The defendants were Stonewall B. Stickney, then Executive Officer of the Alabama State Mental Health Board; Dr. John V. Hottel, his Chief Deputy; the members of the Board; then Governor Albert P. Brewer, both in his capacity as Governor and in his capacity as a member of the Board; and Judge Perry O. Hooper, Probate Judge of Montgomery County, both individually and as a representative of the class consisting of all probate judges in Alabama.

The complaint alleged that the defendants had effected the staff reductions purely for budgetary reasons; that the discharges of the 99 employees had been accomplished without notice and a hearing, and violated the employees' rights under the due process clause; and that as a result of the discharges the patients at Bryce would not receive adequate treatment. The complaint sought injunctive relief requiring the defendants to insure that treatment programs then

---

2. The 99 employees included 41 who were assigned duties such as food service, maintenance, typing and other mechanical duties not involving direct patient care; 26 persons involved in planning social and other recreational activities for the patients; nine persons from the department of psychology; eleven from the social service department; three registered nurses, two physicians, one dentist, and six dental aides.

being administered at Bryce would not be interrupted or altered, and requiring the defendants to rescind the terminations of the 99 employees.

The original complaint did not allege that treatment levels at Bryce had been inadequate before the terminations. For reasons not entirely clear from the record before us, however, the focus of the litigation soon shifted from the effects of the October 1970· terminations to questions of the overall adequacy of the treatment afforded at the Alabama state mental hospitals. On January 4, 1971, the plaintiffs amended the complaint to add prayers that the defendants be enjoined from operating Bryce "in a manner that does not conform to constitutional standards of delivering adequate mental treatment to its patients"; that the Court order defendants to prepare a "comprehensive constitutionally acceptable plan to provide adequate treatment in any state mental health facility"; and that the court declare that patients confined to a state mental health facility are entitled to "adequate, competent treatment".

On March 12, 1971, the district court ruled on the plaintiffs' motion for a preliminary injunction. 325 F.Supp. 781. The court's opinion reflected the shift in the focus of the case. In its opinion, the court declared that patients "involuntarily committed through noncriminal procedures and without the constitutional protections that are afforded defendants in criminal proceedings" are "committed for treatment purposes" and so "unquestionably have a constitutional right to receive such individual treatment as will give each of them a realistic opportunity to be cured or to improve his or her mental condition". 325 F.Supp. at 784. The court found that

the treatment programs in effect before the institution of a staff reorganization then in progress were "scientifically and medically inadequate", failing to "conform to any known minimums established for providing treatment for the mentally ill". *Id.* The court stated that it was not at that time in a position to determine whether the treatment which would be provided after the reorganization was completed would be adequate. Accordingly, the court allowed the defendants ninety days to report progress made in the reorganization plan, and to file with the Court a "specific plan" for the provision of adequate treatment at Bryce. Also in the March 12 order, the court invited the United States, through the Department of Justice and Health, Education and Welfare, to appear as amicus.

On August 4, 1971, the plaintiffs amended their complaint to allege that the Searcy Hospital at Mount Vernon, Alabama, the one other state hospital for the mentally ill in Alabama, and the Partlow State School and Hospital, Alabama's state facility for the mentally retarded, were being operated in a constitutionally impermissible manner.

On September 13, 1971, six months after the March 12 order, the defendants filed their report on proposed standards of adequate treatment and their implementation. Objections to the report were later filed by the plaintiffs and by the United States, as well as by several interested private organizations which had been granted leave to appear as amici.[3]

The court announced its conclusions upon review of the report and the objections to it in an opinion issued December 10, 1971. 334 F.Supp. 1341. In this

---

3. By order entered August 20, 1971, the district court granted the motion filed by the American Civil Liberties Union, the American Orthopsychiatric Association, the American Psychological Association, and the American Association on Mental Deficiency, for leave to appear as amici. In this Court, these amici have been joined by the National

Association for Mental Health, the American Psychiatric Association and the National Association for Retarded Children. The seven have filed a joint brief in this Court.

The district court expressed its gratitude to these organizations for their valuable assistance in this difficult and complex case, 344 F.Supp. 375, 390, and we do so, too.

opinion, the district court held that there are three "fundamental conditions for adequate and effective treatment": a "humane physical and psychological environment"; qualified staff "in numbers sufficient to administer adequate treatment"; and individualized treatment plans. The court held that the reports before it showed "rather conclusively" that the treatment programs at Bryce did not meet any of these conditions. It also noted that conditions at Searcy and Partlow seemed little better. It concluded that the defendants had failed to "formulate minimum medical and constitutional standards for the operation of these institutions". The court scheduled a formal hearing to take evidence necessary to establish standards, and said that after the hearing it, the court, would itself "establish standards and in due course order their implementation".

The court postponed the hearings to give the defendants another opportunity to formulate proposed minimum standards. On January 17, 1972, the parties and *amici* met in Atlanta, Georgia, where they undertook extensive discussions concerning the proper standards of treatment at the Alabama hospitals. Out of these discussions came two Memoranda of Agreement stipulating certain of the standards necessary to define what would constitute minimally adequate mental treatment at a state psychiatric institution. One of the Memoranda covered standards for treatment at the mental hospitals, Searcy and Bryce; the other covered standards to be imposed at the school for the mentally retarded, Partlow. These Memoranda

were filed with the district court at the times for the hearings set for determining the proper standards. The hearing concerning Bryce and Searcy was held February 3 and 4, 1972; the hearing concerning Partlow was held February 28–March 2.[4]

The district court announced its orders granting permanent injunctive relief in two opinions issued April 13, 1972. One of the opinions concerned Partlow, the other, Bryce and Searcy. 344 F.Supp. 373 (Bryce-Searcy), 390 (Partlow). In Partlow, Judge Johnson held that "[b]ecause the only constitutional justification for civilly committing a mental retardate . . . is habilitation, it follows ineluctably" that civilly committed retardates "have a constitutional right to receive such individual habilitation as will give each of them a realistic opportunity to lead a more useful and meaningful life and to return to society". The Bryce-Searcy opinion summarized the court's earlier opinions, noting its holding that the civilly mentally ill have a constitutional right to treatment. Beyond this, the two opinions were substantially identical. Both ordered the defendants (1) to implement an elaborate set of standards of treatment set forth in appendices to the opinions; (2) to establish human rights committees at the institutions to review all research and treatment programs "to ensure that the dignity and human rights of the residents are preserved"; (3) to prepare and file reports within six months of the orders on the implementation of the standards; and (4) to pay court costs and a reasonable attorneys' fee to the plaintiffs. The Partlow

---

4. At the conclusion of the Partlow hearing, the district court entered an emergency order requiring the defendants to take certain immediate actions at Partlow. These included the installation of an emergency light system and procedures for emergency evacuation; revision of sanitation measures in the kitchen; revamping of its program for the use of drugs; conducting appropriate immunizations; and employing three hundred additional resident care workers. In its order

filed March 2, 1972, the court said it was taking these steps "to protect the lives and well-being of the residents", because it found Partlow to be a "warehousing institution . . . wholly incapable of furnishing treatment to the mentally retarded and . . . conducive only to the deterioriation and debilitation of the residents", and because it found conditions at Partlow "substandard to the point of endangering the health and lives of the residents".

order also required the defendants to hire a qualified administrator for the School within sixty days.[5]

Governor Wallace and the Mental Health Board filed separate notices of appeal May 12, 1972. On May 22, Governor Wallace filed a motion for modification and for a stay pending appeal. On June 1, the district court issued an opinion fixing the amount due plaintiffs as attorneys' fees at $36,744.62. 344 F. Supp. at 408–411. On June 26, the district court denied the motions for modification and for a stay pending appeal. This Court also denied a motion for a stay pending appeal.

B. *The conditions in the Alabama hospitals*

There has not been any significant dispute, in this Court or in the district court, about the conditions that prevailed in the Alabama hospitals at the time this suit was instituted. The defendants have pitched their defense on their argument that the Constitution does not guarantee a right to treatment; they have virtually conceded that if such a constitutional right exists, the conditions in the hospitals were such that the state's constitutional obligation to provide adequate treatment could not be met. There is therefore little reason for an extended discussion of the conditions that prevailed at the hospitals. Some discussion, however, is essential to understanding this case. We therefore note briefly how far short the hospitals fell of meeting the three "fundamental conditions of adequate and effective treatment" defined by the district court.

First, it is clear that the environment at the hospitals was a far cry from the "humane psychological and physical environment" the district court envisioned as *sine qua non* of rehabilitative treatment. Bryce Hospital was built in the 1850's; it had 5000 inmates of whom 1500 to 1600 were geriatrics, 1000 were mental retardates, and there were allegedly other non-mentally ill persons. Patients in the hospitals were afforded virtually no privacy: the wards were overcrowded; there was no furniture where patients could keep clothing; there were no partitions between commodes in the bathrooms. There were severe health and safety problems: patients with open wounds and inadequately treated skin diseases were in imminent danger of infection because of the unsanitary conditions existing in the wards, such as permitting urine and feces to remain on the floor; there was evidence of insect infestation in the kitchen and dining areas. Malnutrition was a problem: the United States described the food as "com[ing] closer to 'punishment' by starvation" than nutrition. At Bryce, the food distribution and preparation systems were unsanitary, and less than 50 cents per day per patient was spent on food. Dr. Donald L. Clopper, Associate Commissioner for Mental Retardation for the Alabama Department of Mental Health, testified that Partlow was a "stepchild" in the State of Alabama; that the physical environment was inadequate for treating inmates; that "we don't have the staff we don't have the facilities, nor do we have the financial resources". According to Dr. Clopper, at least 300 Partlow inmates could be discharged immediately, and about 70 percent of the inmates should never have been committed; yet it was 60 percent over-crowded. Patients at Partlow were forced to perform uncompensated labor. Aides frequently put patients in seclu-

---

5. In both orders, the court refused requests made by plaintiffs and amici to appoint a master and professional advisory committee to oversee implementation of the standards on grounds that "[f]ederal courts are reluctant to assume control of any organization, but especially one operated by a state". 344 F.Supp. at 377, 392–393. The court also, in both orders, reserved ruling on various mo-

tions by the plaintiffs to ensure adequate financing for the implementation of the standards. These included a motion that the Mental Health Board be directed to sell or encumber its extensive land holdings, and a motion for an injunction against the expenditure of state funds on any "nonessential" functions until the standards were fully implemented.

sion or under physical restraints, including straitjackets, without physicians' orders. One resident had been regularly confined in a straitjacket for more than nine years. The Evaluation Report on Partlow by the American Association on Mental Deficiency stated that nine working residents would feed 54 young boys ground food from one very large bowl with nine plates and nine spoons; "since there were no accommodations to even sit down to eat," it was impossible to tell which residents had been fed and which had not been fed with this system. Seclusion rooms were large enough for one bed and a coffee can, which served as a toilet. The patients suffered brutality, both at the hands of the aides and at the hands of their fellow patients; testimony established that four Partlow residents died due to understaffing, lack of supervision, and brutality.[6]

The hospitals failed to meet the second condition, adequate staffing. The defendants' chief witness on standards maintained that treatment could be delivered with the ratio of one psychiatrist, one graduate level psychologist, and one masters level social worker for every 125 patients, and the district court ultimately adopted this recommendation. The organizations appearing as amici had recommended higher ratios—one psychiatrist, one psychologist, and one social worker for every 30–50 patients. But at the time this suit was instituted there were ratios of only one medical doctor with some psychiatric training for 5,000 patients, one Ph.D. psychologist for every 1,670 patients, and one masters level social worker for every 2,500 patients at Bryce. The parties and amici agreed completely on the minimums necessary for treatment of the mentally retarded. They agreed that adequate treatment could be delivered at Partlow with ratios of one masters level

psychologist and one masters level social worker for every sixty patients, and one physician for every two hundred patients. Yet at Partlow there were only one psychologist with masters level training or above for every 1,200 patients; one masters level social worker for every 730 patients; and one physician for every 550 patients. Of the four physicians at Partlow, two were not licensed to practice in Alabama.

A severe shortage of nonprofessional staff paralleled the inadequacies of professional staff. After a tour of Bryce, defendants' own consultants noted that:

> Aide staff is spread very thin, creating extreme stresses for individual aides, who at times must cover one or two or three wards, housing as many as 100 or 200 patients. Obviously, it is impossible under such circumstances to provide anything more than a cursory observation and the hope of avoiding disturbing incidents. An aide under these circumstances is hard pressed to meet even minimum patient needs.

The institutional staff was inadequate not only in sheer numbers but also in training; there was no effective "inservice training" program for, or even any regular supervision over, the nonprofessionals.

Finally, the evidence established that the hospitals failed to meet the third condition, individualized treatment programs. According to one consultant's testimony, care of patients at Partlow was not suited to the needs of particular individuals, but was instead "geared primarily to housekeeping functions—cleaning floors, cleaning beds, cleaning patients—and to a continuation of work assignments". Experts testified that the patient records kept at the hospital were wholly inadequate; that they were written in such a way as to be incompre-

---

6. One of the four died after a garden hose had been inserted into his rectum for five minutes by a working patient who was cleaning him; one died when a fellow patient hosed him with scalding water; another died when soapy water was forced into his mouth; and a fourth died from a self-administered overdose of drugs which had been inadequately secured.

hensible to the aide level staff that had prime responsibility for patient care; and that they were kept where they were not accessible to the direct care staff particularly in need of them.

II.

[1] The appellants' first and principal contention on appeal is that the Constitution does not guarantee persons civilly committed to state mental institutions a right to treatment.[7] This contention is largely foreclosed by our decision, issued since the institution of this appeal, in Donaldson v. O'Connor, 1974, 493 F.2d 507. In *Donaldson*, we held that civilly committed mental patients have a constitutional right to such individual treatment as will help each of them to be cured or to improve his or her mental condition. We reasoned that the only permissible justifications for civil commitment, and for the massive abridgments of constitutionally protected liberties it entails, were the danger posed by the individual committed to himself or to others, or the individual's need for treatment and care. We held that where the justification for commitment was treatment, it offended the fundamentals of due process if treatment were not in fact provided; and we held that where the justification was the danger to self or to others, then treat-

ment had to be provided as the *quid pro quo* society had to pay as the price of the extra safety it derived from the denial of individuals' liberty.

Our discussion in *Donaldson*, briefly summarized here, answers most of the arguments made by the appellants on this appeal against the recognition of a constitutional right to treatment. Governor Wallace, however, makes one argument not answered by our discussion in *Donaldson*, and it is appropriate that we address that argument here. Governor Wallace challenged the assumption, made by the district court in this case and by this Court in *Donaldson*, that the only permissible justifications for confinement are danger to self or others or need for treatment. Instead, the Governor suggests, the principal justification for commitment lies in the inability of the mentally ill and mentally retarded to care for themselves. The essence of this argument is that the primary function of civil commitment is to relieve the burden imposed upon the families and friends of the mentally disabled. The families and friends of the disabled, the Governor asserts, are the "true clients" of the institutionalization system.[8]

From this premise the Governor proceeds to the conclusion that is the crux of his argument. If "need for care" is a justification for commitment—or is *the*

---

7. In raising the issue in this Court, the appellants contend that, because there is no constitutional right to treatment, the district court lacked jurisdiction over the suit. In so arguing the issue, the appellants are following, on this point as one the other four of their first five contentions, the decision of the Northern District of Georgia in Burnham v. Department of Public Health, 1972, 349 F.Supp. 1335, appeal docketed, No. 72–3110, 5 Cir., Oct. 4, 1972. In *Burnham*, the court held that the Constitution does not guarantee a right to treatment. It then held that the consequence of this conclusion was that it was without jurisdiction over the suit, because 28 U.S.C. § 1343(3), the asserted basis of jurisdiction, confers jurisdiction only over "action[s] . . . to redress the deprivation" of a "right, privilege, or immunity" secured by the Constitution or by an Act of Congress providing for equal rights.

8. Governor Wallace borrows the term "true clients" from the work of Professor Erving Goffman. E. Goffman, Asylums—Essays on the Social Situations of Mental Patients and Other Inmates 384 (1961). Governor Wallace in his brief praises Professor Goffman as a "realistic writer". Be that as it may, it is fairly clear that Professor Goffman's intent, in calling "relatives, police, and judges" the "true clients" of the mental hospitals" was critical, indeed harshly so, and that Professor Goffman was insinuating by that statement an embarrassing, though rarely admitted, truth about the institutionalization system in the United States. What Professor Goffman implied was morally unacceptable—that the convenience of relatives and law enforcers justifies stripping away all of the liberties of the civilly committed —we hold today is constitutionally unacceptable.

justification—then it follows that the mere provision of custodial care is constitutionally adequate to justify continued confinement. "[T]he providing of custodial care alone is a tremendously important consideration to patients, their families, and the public-at-large", the Governor writes in his brief.

There are two answers to this line of argument. The first, and more limited, is that even accepting the Governor's premise that "need for care" is a constitutionally adequate justification for confinement, it does not follow that we must accept the conclusion—that *the kind of care that was provided at the Alabama hospitals* is sufficient to make continued confinement constitutional. The assertion that "need for care" justifies confinement implies that the state has an affirmative obligation to provide a certain minimum quality "care", no less than the assertion that "need for treatment" justifies confinement implies that the state has an affirmative obligation to provide a certain minimum quality "treatment". And it is clear that, however that obligation might specifically be defined, it was not being met in the Alabama hospitals. Dr. Gunnar Dybwad, Professor of Human Development at the Graduate School for Advanced Studies in Social Welfare at Brandeis University, and a one time presidential consultant in the field of mental retardation, made essentially this point when he testified about conditions at Alabama's Partlow State School and Hospital:

> The situation which exists and obviously has existed in Partlow for a long time is one of storage, of persons. I am using that word because *I would not use care, which involves*—has a certain qualitative character, and *I would not even use the word, 'custodial,' because custody, in my term, means safekeeping.* And, as is visible to the visitor at the present time, employees at Partlow are *not in a position to effect safekeeping,* considering the number of people they have to take care of; so I would say it is a

storage problem at the moment. (Emphasis supplied.)

Indeed, many of the standards established by the district court in this case —notably those required for what the district court called a "humane psychological and physical environment"— might have to be met for the state to be able legitimately to claim it was providing adequate "care" to its mental patients. At least where the right to a "humane environment" is concerned, then if it is irrelevant whether the right be viewed as a facet of a "right to treatment", or of a "right to care". It is likewise irrelevant for those purposes whether the state interest imputed to the civil commitment system be called the need "to treat" the mentally ill, or the need "to care" for them.

[2] But beyond this, we find it impossible to accept the Governor's underlying premise that the "need to care" for the mentally ill—and to relieve their families, friends, or guardians of the burdens of doing so—can supply a constitutional justification for civil commitment. At stake in the civil commitment context, as we emphasized in *Donaldson,* see 493 F.2d at 520, are "massive curtailments" of individual liberty. Against the sweeping personal interests involved, Governor Wallace would have us weigh the state's interest, and the interests of the friends and families of the mentally handicapped in having private parties relieved of the "burden" of caring for the mentally ill. The state interest thus asserted may be, strictly speaking, a "rational" state interest. But we find it so trivial beside the major personal interests against which it is to be weighed that we cannot possibly accept it as a justification for the deprivations of liberty involved.

The other arguments against recognition of a constitutional right to treatment for civilly committed mental patients advanced by the appellants are, as we noted above, answered by our discussion in *Donaldson.* Following *Donaldson,* we hold that the district court here did not err in finding that civilly committed mental patients have a constitutional right to treatment. Our express holding in *Donaldson* and here rests on the *quid pro quo* concept of "rehabilitative treatment, or, where rehabilitation is impossible, minimally adequate habilitation and care, beyond the subsistence level custodial care that would be provided in a penitentiary." 493 F.2d at 522.

III.

[3] The second, third, fourth, and fifth issues raised by the appellants are also substantially affected by our decision in *Donaldson,* and present little difficulty except as to some aspects of remedy which will be discussed in Part IV, infra. The argument that this suit is barred by the eleventh amendment is based largely upon Burnham v. Department of Public Health, N.D.Ga.1972, 349 F.Supp. 1335, appeal docketed, No. 72–3110, 5 Cir., Oct. 4, 1972, a case consolidated for argument on appeal with this case. In *Burnham,* the court held that, because the right to treatment was a right arising only, if at all, under state law, a suit by citizens of the state against state officials to enforce the right was barred by the eleventh amendment. Our holding in *Donaldson,* however, vitiates this argument, of course, for we have now established that the right to treatment arises as a matter of federal constitutional law under the due process clause of the Fourteenth Amendment.

[4] In *Donaldson,* we addressed and rejected the argument that a constitutional right to adequate treatment would present questions not susceptible to "judicially manageable or ascertainable standards". We held that the judiciary was competent to determine, at least in individual cases, whether psychiatric treatment was medically or constitutionally adequate. And we said in dictum that even in cases such as this one, "when courts are asked to undertake the more difficult task of fashioning institution-wide standards of adequacy", 493 F.2d at 526, the courts would be able to formulate workable standards. In *Donaldson,* we took note of the substantial agreement reached in this case among parties and *amici* in developing standards during the course of the proceedings in the lower court. We cited that development as evidence supporting our view that workable standards could be fashioned. We remain mindful of that development here, in reaffirming our belief that the right to treatment can be implemented through judicially manageable standards.

[5] The appellants' fourth contention is that the order of the district court invades a province of decision-making exclusively reserved for the state legislature. Governor Wallace argues that the order will require heavy expenditures of state funds; that these funds will have to come from other state programs; and that the duty of compromising and allocating funds among the many programs competing for them is a duty which must be discharged by the state governor and legislature alone. Governor Wallace concedes in his brief that he is not contending that "the financial cost of complying with an established constitutional right is a valid reason for failure to comply". He "suggest[s] that before the Court decides to adopt a new constitutional right it should consider all of the consequences of its action, financial and social, and its effect on our federal form of government". The Mental Health Board makes the point in a related way, by suggesting that the district court's order here is in effect an order requiring the state to furnish a particular service, and by citing cases establishing the general proposition that ordinarily it is· not for the federal courts to say whether or in what amounts a state shall provide any particular government benefit or service. *E. g.,* Fullington v. Shea, D.Colo.1970, 320 F.Supp. 500, aff'd, 404 U.S. 963, 92 S.Ct. 345, 30 L.Ed.2d 282.

We find these arguments unpersuasive. It goes without saying that state legislatures are ordinarily free to choose among various social services competing for legislative attention and state funds. But that does not mean that a state legislature is free, for budgetary or any other reasons, to provide a social service in a manner which will result in the denial of individuals' constitutional rights. And it is the essence of our holding, here and in *Donaldson*, that the provision of treatment to those the state has involuntarily confined in mental hospitals is necessary to make the state's actions in confining and continuing to confine those individuals constitutional. That being the case, the state may not fail to provide treatment for budgetary reasons alone. "Humane considerations and constitutional requirements are not, in this day, to be measured or limited by dollar considerations". Jackson v. Bishop, 8 Cir. 1968, 404 F.2d 571, 580 (Blackmun, J.), quoted, Rozecki v. Gaughan, 1 Cir. 1972, 459 F.2d 6, 8. "Inadequate resources can never be an adequate justification for the state's depriving any person of his constitutional rights". Hamilton v. Love, E.D.Ark. 1972, 328 F.Supp. 1182, 1194. "[T]he obligation of the Respondents [prison officials] to eliminate unconstitutionalities does not depend upon what the Legislatures may do". Holt v. Sarver, E.D.Ark.1970, 309 F.Supp. 362, 385, aff'd, 8 Cir. 1971, 442 F.2d 304. See also Hawkins v. Town of Shaw, 5 Cir. 1971, 437 F.2d 1286, 1292.

This conclusion is not novel. In the context of state penal institutions, the federal courts have repeatedly intervened to assure that the conditions of confinement do not invade the constitutional rights of those confined. E. g., Cruz v. Beto, 1972, 405 U.S. 319, 92 S. Ct. 1079, 31 L.Ed.2d 263; Johnson v. Avery, 1968, 393 U.S. 483, 89 S.Ct. 747, 21 L.Ed.2d 718; Campbell v. Beto, 5 Cir. 1972, 460 F.2d 765; Landman v. Royster, E.D.Va.1971, 333 F.Supp. 621; Holt v. Sarver, E.D.Ark.1970, 309 F. Supp. 362, aff'd, 8 Cir. 1971, 442 F. 2d 304. This Court has recognized that "our constitutional duties require that the courts be ever vigilant to assure that the conditions of incarceration do

not overstep the bounds of federal constitutional limitations". *Campbell*, 460 F.2d at 767–768. In discharging these duties, the federal courts have in some cases entered decrees requiring substantial restructuring of state prison systems, but the courts have not hesitated to enter such decrees when necessary to safeguard the constitutional rights of prisoners. As the court said in Holt v. Sarver:

Let there be no mistake in the matter; the obligation of the Respondents to eliminate existing unconstitutionalities does not depend upon what the Legislature may do, or upon what the Governor may do, or, indeed, upon what Respondents may actually be able to accomplish. If Arkansas is going to operate a Penitentiary System, it is going to have to be a system that is countenanced by the Constitution of the United States.

309 F.Supp. at 385.

Similar developments have occurred in the field of institutions for the detention of juveniles. Nelson v. Heyne, 7 Cir. 1974, 491 F.2d 352, aff'g, N.D.Ind. 1972, 355 F.Supp. 451; Martarella v. Kelley, S.D.N.Y.1972, 359 F.Supp. 479, enforcing, 349 F.Supp. 575; Inmates of Boys' Training School v. Affleck, D.R.I. 1972, 346 F.Supp. 1354; Morales v. Turman, E.D.Tex.1973, 364 F.Supp. 166.

[6] The appellants' fifth contention, that the plaintiffs had adequate remedies at law, is also unpersuasive. In the *Burnham* case, the court held that the legal remedies of "habeas corpus, medical malpractice, and ordinary tort actions" would supply adequate remedies to mental patients who claimed to have been denied a right to treatment. 349 F.Supp. at 1343. It found the plaintiffs' arguments to the contrary "inconsistent with plaintiffs argument that each individual patient should have his particular therapy or treatment personalized". *Id.* Governor Wallace and the Mental Health Board urge here the argument that damage and habeas corpus actions provide adequate legal remedies to the plaintiffs. They also point to the

plaintiffs' argument that treatment must be individualized, and to the tension between that argument and the plaintiffs' insistence that injunctive relief on behalf of the plaintiff class is appropriate in this case.

We are unable to agree that injunctive relief is inappropriate merely because damages or habeas corpus relief may be available to some or all individual plaintiffs. While habeas corpus and tort remedies should play a valuable, indeed essential, role in enforcing the constitutional rights we recognized in *Donaldson*, those remedies are not capable of ensuring what the plaintiffs seek to ensure in this case. In the first place, habeas corpus relief and tort damages are available only after the fact of a failure to provide individual treatment. Here the plaintiffs seek preventive relief, to assure in advance that mental patients will at least have the *chance* to receive adequate treatment by proscribing the maintenance of conditions that foredoom *all* mental patients *inevitably* to inadequate mental treatment. Moreover, there are special reasons why reliance upon individual suits by mental patients would be especially inappropriate. Mental patients are particularly unlikely to be aware of their legal rights. They are likely to have especially limited access to legal assistance. Individual suits may be protracted and expensive, and individual mental patients may therefore be deterred from bringing them. And individual suits may produce distortive therapeutic effects within an institution, since a staff may tend to give especially good—or especially harsh—treatment to patients the staff expects or knows to be litigious.[9]

We see no inconsistency between this conclusion and the position taken by the plaintiffs, and by the district court, that treatment must be individualized. The plaintiffs here do not seek to *guarantee* that all patients will receive all the treatment they need or that may be appropriate to them. They seek only to ensure that conditions in the state institutions will be such that the patients confined there will have a *chance* to receive adequate treatment. This requires only the establishment of a program, institution-wide in scope, for developing and formulating individual treatment plans; it of course does not require the formulation, in this suit, of each individual plan. The question of what is necessary to the establishment of such a program is better resolved in a class action brought on behalf of all patients than it would be in a series of individual suits.

IV.

We pretermit decision as to the remedy decreed by the district court to the extent herein stated. As we have held, the legislative power may not be used to deprive appellees of their constitutional right to treatment, but a substantial question is presented as to the scope of judicial power in implementing this right. The ultimate question will be, if all else fails, the method of effecting the financial outlay which will be necessary for the judiciary to give meaning to judicially prescribed minimum constitutional standards for adequate treatment of the mentally ill.

Prior to the entry of the court's orders on April 13, 1972, 344 F.Supp. 373; 344 F.Supp. 387, the parties and amici stipulated to a number of specific conditions they agreed were necessary for a constitutionally acceptable minimum treatment program.[10] Because of these stipulations, we need not and do not

9. See 86 Harv.L.Rev. 1282, 1305 (1973).

10. The parties and amici submitted in two Memoranda of Agreement stipulations of standards of adequate care. Virtually all of the specifics of the district court's April 13, 1972 orders were taken from these stipulations. These standards have not been challenged on appeal. Indeed, Governor Wallace's brief to this court begins with the affirmation: "We wish to emphasize at the outset that this appellant, Governor George C. Wallace, is in full and complete agreement with the ultimate achievement of the standards and goals for mental health facilities which are set forth in the District Court's order[s] of April 13, 1972." Brief of Appellant, p. 1.

reach decision as to whether the standards prescribed by the district court are constitutionally minimum requirements, or whether it is within the province of a federal district court, three-judge or single judge, to prescribe standards as distinguished from enjoining the operation of such institutions while constitutional rights are being violated.

[7]   Governor Wallace contends such stipulations are not binding on him or the Alabama legislature. As a party to the stipulations, through counsel, we hold the Governor has for his part agreed that these standards are minimally acceptable under the Constitution. The Alabama legislature presents a different problem. Clearly the Governor is without authority to agree to the expenditure of funds required to implement such a broad spectrum of standards when such a decision under Alabama law is reserved to the legislature. That the legislature was not a party to the stipulations in question or to this law suit reenforces this manifest principle of governmental organization. It is the Governor's role to propose relief to the legislature and, having stipulated the standards, to use his best efforts to accomplish the relief.

With respect to judicial accomplishment of the remedy, profound questions are presented regarding the scope of substantive due process and the role of federal courts in matters affecting the management of state institutions. Here we are concerned with the operation of state mental institutions within the parameters of substantive due process.[11]

[8]   The governor argues that the prescribed remedy will entail the expenditure annually of a sum equal to sixty per cent of the state budget excluding school financing, and a capital improvements outlay of $75,000,000. This is contested by appellees. However that may be, we regard as premature any issue as to whether the district court should appoint a Special Master for the purposes of selling or encumbering state lands to finance these standards, or should enjoin certain state officials from authorizing expenditures for nonessential state functions, and thereby alter the state budget, or by other means order a particular mode of financing the implementation of the stipulated standards.

Such remedial propositions are by the terms of the district court's April 13, 1972 not present orders; they lie in the uncertain future. The district court wrote:

".   .   . this Court has decided to reserve ruling also upon plaintiffs' motion that defendant Mental Health Board be directed to sell or encumber portions of its land holdings in order to raise funds. Similarly, this Court will reserve ruling on plaintiffs' motion seeking an injunction against the treasurer and the comptroller of the State authorizing expenditures for nonessential State functions, and on other aspects of plaintiffs' requested

---

11. As noted, supra, however rare thay may be, federal decrees mandating affirmative action expenditures by state governing authorities to ensure constitutional guarantees are not unprecedented in cases involving equal protection and also cruel and unusual punishment. *E. g.*, Griffin v. County School Bd., 1964, 377 U.S. 218, 233, 84 S.Ct. 1226, 12 L.Ed.2d 256, 266; Swann v. Charlotte-Mecklenburg Md. of Educ., N.D.N.C., 1970, 311 F.Supp. 265, 268, vacated and remanded on other grounds, 4 Cir. (en banc), 431 F.2d 138, order reinstated, 1971, 402 U.S. 1, 91 S. Ct. 1267, 28 L.Ed.2d 554 ; United States v. Plaquemines Parish School Bd., E.D.La., 1967, 291 F.Supp. 841, aff'd as modified, 5 Cir., 1969, 415 F.2d 817; Cruz v. Beto, 1972, 405 U.S. 319, 92 S.Ct. 1079, 31 L. Ed.2d 263; Holt v. Sarver, 8 Cir., 1971, 442 F.2d 304; Nelson v. Heyne, 7 Cir., 1974, 491 F.2d 352; Gautreaux v. Chicago Housing Auth., N.D.Ill., 1969, 296 F.Supp. 907, aff'd, 7 Cir., 1970, 436 F.2d 306, cert. denied, 1971, 402 U.S. 922, 91 S.Ct. 1378, 28 L.Ed.2d 661.
See also cases cited Note, Right To Treatment, 1973, 86 Harv.L.Rev. 1282, 1300, nn. 98–104; Developments in the Law, Civil Commitment of the Mentally Ill, 1974, 87 Harv.L.Rev. 1338, n. 96; Comment, Enforcement of Judicial Financing Order; Constitutional Rights in Search of a Remedy, 1970, 59 Geo.L.J. 393.

relief designed to ameliorate the financial problems incident to the implementation of this order. . . . The responsibility for appropriate funding ultimately must fall, of course, upon the State Legislature and, to a lesser degree, upon the defendant Mental Health Board of Alabama. For the present time, the Court will defer to those bodies in hopes that they will proceed with the realization and understanding that what is involved in this case is not representative of ordinary governmental functions such as paving roads and maintaining buildings. Rather, what is so inextricably intertwined with how the Legislature and Mental Health Board respond to the revelations of this litigation is the very preservation of human life and dignity . . .

In the event, though, that the Legislature fails to satisfy its well-defined constitutional obligation, and the Mental Health Board, because of lack of funding or any other legally insufficient reason, fails to implement fully the standards herein ordered, it will be necessary for the Court to take affirmative steps, including appointing a master, to ensure that proper funding is realized and that adequate treatment is available for the mentally ill in Alabama." 344 F.Supp. at 377–378. See also 344 F.Supp. at 393–394. (These separate orders cover the three institutions involved.)

To the latter statement, the district court added in a footnote, 344 F.Supp. at 378, n. 8:

"The Court understands and appreciates that the Legislature is not due back in regular session until May, 1973. Nevertheless, special sessions of the Legislature are frequent occurrences in Alabama, and there has never been a time when such a session was more urgently required. If the Legislature does not act promptly to appropriate the necessary funding for mental health, the Court will be compelled to grant plaintiffs' motion to add various State officials and agencies as additional parties to this litigation, and to utilize other avenues of fund raising." See also 344 F.Supp. at 394, n. 14.

The district court ordered that defendants file within six months a detailed report on the implementation of the stipulated standards.

The serious constitutional questions presented by federal judicial action ordering the sale of state lands, or altering the state budget, or which may otherwise arise in the problem of financing, in the event the governing authorities fail to move in good faith to ensure what all parties agree are minimal requirements, should not be adjudicated unnecessarily and prematurely. *See* Ashwander v. Tennessee Valley Authority, 1936, 297 U.S. 288, 346–348, 56 S.Ct. 466, 80 L.Ed. 688, 710–712 (Brandeis, J., concurring); *cf.* Hawkins v. Town of Shaw, 5 Cir. (en banc), 1972, 461 F.2d 1171; Holt v. Sarver, 8 Cir., 1971, 442 F.2d 304, 309. Since we have now affirmed that part of the district court's orders recognizing the constitutional right to treatment, determination of good faith efforts by state authorities to ensure these rights should be made in the first instance in the district court.

[9] In any event, as a jurisdictional matter dictated by federal statute, remedies of the type contemplated in the district court order of April 13, 1972 are required to be determined by a district court of three judges. Any federal decree that state lands be sold or legislative appropriations be reallocated or enjoined would involve state laws of statewide significance within the purview of 28 U.S.C.A. § 2281. The federal injunctive decree which might be entered in such circumstances is required to be that of a three-judge district court. Sands v. Wainwright, *supra*, 491 F.2d 417. We of course make no prejudg-

ment as to the appropriateness of any such remedial order. Moreover, depending on the improvements made or in progress, such remedies may be unnecessary.

This court views as serious a state's failure to ensure the fulfillment of appellees' constitutional rights, but the interests of all concerned, and the sensitivities of our federal system, will be best served by the parties, amici, and court moving together to meet the constitutional requisites. This is the nature of the remedy ordered by this court in Hawkins v. Town of Shaw, *supra*, 461 F.2d at 1174. This appears to be the meaning and intent of the district court's recognition of the function of the Alabama legislature within the Alabama governmental framework, and the court's orders of April 13, 1972 requiring reports on compliance with the stipulated standards.

This approach should hasten the day when the district court can be reasonably assured that appellees' constitutional rights are no longer being violated, and when ultimate control over the institutions in question can be returned to the state. *Cf.* Holt v. Sarver, *supra*, 442 F.2d at 309.

V.

We reserve decision on the issue presented by the awards of attorneys' fees to plaintiffs pending decision in No. 73–1790, Gates v. Collier; No. 73–2033, Newman v. State of Alabama; and Named Individual Members of the San Antonio Conservation Society v. Texas Highway Department, en banc, argued and submitted on October 2, 1974. See 28 U.S.C.A. § 2106 for the authority to reserve decision.

Affirmed in part; remanded in part for further proceedings not inconsistent herewith; and decision reserved in part.

Wyatt v. Hardin

Ricky WYATT, by and through his aunt and legal guardian, Mrs. W. C. Rawlins, Jr., et al., Plaintiffs,

v.

Taylor HARDIN, as Commissioner of Mental Health and the State of Alabama Mental Health Officer, et al., Defendants.

United States of America et al., Amici Curiae.

Civ. A. No. 3195-N

United States District Court,
M.D. Alabama, N.D.

February 28, 1975

ORDER

Pursuant to this Court's direction of October 1, 1974, the parties and *amici curiae* have filed written responses to the suggestions of defendants and the Searcy Human Rights Committee that Standard 9[1] of this Court's order of April 13, 1972, be modified. After a thorough considera-

---

[1]"Patients have a right not to be subjected to treatment procedures such as lobotomy, electro-convulsive treatment, adversive reinforcement conditioning or other unusual or hazardous treatment procedures without their express and informed consent after consultation with counsel or interested party of the patient's choice." *Wyatt* v. *Stickney,* 344 F. Supp. 373, 380 (M.D. Ala. 1972), *aff'd* 503 F.2d 1305 (5th Cir. 1974).

tion of these written requests and responses and the Court's further study of Bryce and Searcy hospitals' experiences in operating under Standard 9, the Court is of the opinion that a substantial revision of the present Standard 9 is in order.

It must be emphasized at the outset of this order that, in setting forth the minimum constitutional requirements for the employment of certain extraordinary or potentially hazardous modes of treatment, the Court is not undertaking to determine which forms of treatment are appropriate in particular situations. Such a diagnostic decision is a medical judgment and is not within the province, jurisdiction or expertise of this Court. But the determination of what procedural safeguards must accompany the use of extraordinary or potentially hazardous modes of treatment on patients in the state's mental institutions is a fundamentally legal question and one which the parties to this lawsuit have put at issue.

Accordingly, it is ORDERED that Standard 9 of the April 13, 1972, order in this cause be and is hereby rescinded.

It is further ORDERED that the following standards be and they are hereby adopted and ordered implemented from this date:

1. No lobotomy, psychosurgery or other unusual, hazardous or intrusive surgical procedure designed to alter or affect a patient's mental condition shall be performed on any patient confined at any institution maintained by or under the control of the defendants.

2. No patient shall be subjected to any aversive conditioning or other systematic attempt to alter his behavior by means of painful or noxious stimuli, except under the floowing conditions:

a. A program of aversive conditioning has been recommended by a Qualified Mental Health Professional trained and experienced in the use of aversive conditioning. This recommendation shall be made in writing with detailed clinical justification and an explanation of which alternative treatments were considered and why they were rejected. The recommendation must be concurred in by another Qualified Mental Health Professional trained and experienced in the use of aversive conditioning and approved by the superintendent or medical director of the hospital.

b. Any program of aversive therapy proposed for the benefit of an institution's patients shall have first been reviewed and approved by that institution's Human Rights Committee before its use shall be recommended by a Qualified Mental Health Professional for an individual patient.

c. The patient has given his express and informed consent in writing to the administration of aversive conditioning. It shall be the responsibility of the treating psychiatrist to provide the patient with complete and accurate information concerning the nature and effects of aversive therapy, to assist the patient in comprehending the significance of such information, and to identify any barriers to such comprehension. The written consent signed by the patient shall include a statement of the nature of the treatment consented to; a description of its purpose, risks, and possible effects; and a notice to the patient that he has the right to terminate his consent at any time and for any reason.

d. No aversive conditioning shall be imposed on any patient without the prior approval of the Extraordinary Treatment Committee, formed in accordance with this paragraph, whose primary responsibility it is to determine, after appropriate inquiry and interview with the patient, whether the patient's consent to such therapy is, in fact, knowing, intelligent, and voluntary and whether the proposed treatment is in the best interest of the patient. The Extraordinary Treatment Committee shall consist of five members to be nominated by the Human Rights Committee of the hospital and appointed by the Court. The members shall be so selected that the committee will be competent to deal with the medical, psychological, psychiatric, legal, social and ethical issues involved in such treatment methods; to this end, at least one member shall be a psychiatrist licensed to practice in this state; at least one member shall be a neurologist or a specialist in internal medicine; and at least one member shall be an attorney licensed to practice law in this state. No member shall be an officer, employee or agent of the Department of Mental Health; nor may any member be otherwise involved in the proposed treatment.

e. The patient shall be represented throughout all proceedings, including the signing of his consent and the deliberations of the Extraordinary Treatment Committee, by legal counsel appointed by the Extraordinary Treatment Committee from a list of such counsel compiled by the Human Rights Committee and approved by the Court. Counsel shall assure, *inter alia,* that all considerations militating against the use of aversive conditioning have been adequately explored and resolved and that the patient is competent to consent to such treatment. No such counsel may be an officer, employee or agent of the Department of Mental Health; nor may such counsel be otherwise involved in the proposed treatment.

f. The Extraordinary Treatment Committee shall maintain written records of its approvals and disapprovals of patient consent to aversive conditioning and the reasons therefor, with supporting documentation. Such records shall be available for examination by the hospital Human Rights Committee, the Court, and counsel of record in this cause.

g. Aversive conditioning shall be administered only under the direct supervision of and in the physical presence of a Qualified Mental Health Professional trained and experienced in the use of aversive conditioning.

h. No patient shall be subjected to an aversive conditioning program which attempts to extinguish or alter socially appropriate behavior or to develop new behavior patterns for the sole or primary purpose of institutional convenience.

i. A patient may withdraw his consent to aversive conditioning at any time and for any reason. Such withdrawal of consent may be either oral or written and is to be given effect immediately.

3. No patient shall be subjected to electro-convulsive therapy (ECT), except under the following conditions:

a. The patient is eighteen years of age or older.

b. A program of electro-convulsive therapy is recommended by a Qualified Mental Health Professional trained and experienced in the use of ECT. This recommendation shall be made in writing with detailed clinical justification and an explanation of which alternative treatments were considered and why they were rejected. The recommendation must be concurred in by another Qualified Mental Health Professional trained and experienced in the use of ECT and approved by the superintendent or medical director of the hospital.

c. Express and informed consent to the administration of ECT has been given in writing by the patient, if he is deemed competent to give such consent by the attorney appointed to represent him, the treating psychiatrist, and the Extraordinary Treatment Committee. It shall be the responsibility of the treating psychiatrist to provide the patient with complete and accurate information concerning the nature, risks, and consequences of ECT; to assist the patient in comprehending the significance of such information; and to identify any barriers to such comprehension. The written consent signed by the patient shall include a statement of the nature of the treatment consented to; a description of its purpose, risks, and possible consequences; and a notice to the patient that he has the right to terminate his consent at any time and for any reason.

d. ECT shall not be administered to a patient who has signed a written consent thereto without the prior approval of the Extraordinary Treatment Committee, whose responsibility it is to determine, after appropriate inquiry and interview with the patient, whether his consent to such therapy is, in fact, knowing, intelligent, and voluntary and whether the proposed treatment is the least drastic alternative available for the treatment of his illness.

e. In the event that the patient is deemed incompetent to consent to ECT by either his attorney, the treating psychiatrist or the Extraordinary Treatment Committee, the Committee may consent to such treatment in his behalf if it determines that the evidence presented to it clearly indicates that the administration of ECT is in the patient's best interest. Such a determination shall be based upon:

(1) A review of pertinent medical, psychiatric, psychological, and social information concerning the patient;

(2) The written recommendation of the Qualified Mental Health Professional prepared pursuant to paragraph 3-b above;

(3) An interview with the patient, unless he is physically or emotionally incapable of being interviewed; and

(4) Interviews with members of the patient's family, the hospital staff, and others who in the committee's judgment may contribute relevant information.

The Extraordinary Treatment Committee shall give great weight to any expression by the patient of a desire not to be subjected to ECT. Any doubts that ECT is in the best interest of the incompetent patient shall be resolved against proceeding with such treatment.

f. If the committee concludes that ECT is in the patient's best interest, the patient or any interested member of his family shall have the right to seek review of that determination in a court of competent jurisdiction. If he, or a member of his family or his attorney shall indicate an intention to seek such review, no ECT treatments shall be commenced or continued unless and until authorized by the court to which the matter is presented.

g. The patient shall be represented throughout all proceedings, including the signing of any consent and the deliberations of the Extraordinary Treatment Committee, by legal counsel appointed by the Extraordinary Treatment Committee from a list of such counsel compiled by the Human Rights Committee and approved by the Court. Counsel shall assure, *inter alia,* that all considerations militating against the use of electro-convulsive therapy have been adequately explored and resolved and that the proposed treatment has been validly consented to either by the patient or by the Extraordinary Treatment Committee in his behalf. No such counsel may be an officer, employee or agent of the Department of Mental Health; nor may such counsel be otherwise involved in the proposed treatment.

h. the Extraordinary Treatment Committee shall maintain written records of its determinations and the reasons therefor, with supporting documentation. Such records shall be available for examination by the hospital's Human Rights Committee, the Court, and counsel of record in this cause. The Committee shall report in writing at least monthly to the Human Rights Committee, the Court, and counsel of record as to the number of patients approved and disapproved for ECT, the procedures employed in approving or disapproving such treatments, the reasons for such decisions, and any other pertinent information.

i. A complete physical examination, including neurological examination, shall be given to the patient within ten (10) days prior to the commencement of each series of electro-convulsive treatments.

j. ECT shall be administered only by a psychiatrist who is a Qualified Mental Health Professional trained and experienced in the use of ECT or by qualified personnel acting under the direct supervision and in the physical presence of such trained psychiatrist. Anesthesia shall be administered by a qualified anesthetist or anesthesiologist.

k. Anesthesia and muscle relaxants shall be administered in conjunction with ECT unless medically contraindicated.

l. Regressive, multiple or depatterning electro-convulsive techniques shall not be utilized.

m. Prior approval shall be obtained from the Extraordinary Treatment Committee by the treating psychiatrist if more than twelve (12) treatments in one ECT series are recommended for a patient or if more than one series is recommended during any twelve-month period.

n. A competent patient may withdraw his consent to ECT at any time and for any reason. A patient who is incompetent at the inception of a course of treatment may refuse to participate in further treatments at any time that he is restored to competence. Such withdrawal of consent or refusal to participate may be either oral or written and is to be given effect immediately.

4. No patient at any institution maintained by or under the control of the defendants shall be subjected to any other extraordinary or hazardous technique or procedure not specifically mentioned herein unless the treating psychiatrist or the medical director of the hospital has first obtained:

a. The written approval of the Extraordinary Treatment Commitee to the utilization of such technique or procedure; and

b. The express and informed consent of the patient in writing to the administration of such treatment.

5. There shall be no coercion in any form with regard to the treatment of any patient by means of any of the extraordinary techniques dealt with herein. Consent to any such form of treatment shall not be made a condition for receiving any type of public assistance, nor may it be a prerequisite to any health or social service or for admission to or release from any institution maintained by or under the control of the defendants.

6. Complete, accurate, and contemporaneous records shall be maintained with respect to each administration of aversive conditioning or electro-convulsive therapy. Such records shall include, by way of illustration and not of limitation, the date and time of each treatment; the name(s) of the person(s) administering such treatment; the duration of the treatment; a clinical description of the procedure followed; the dosage and identity of any medication prescribed; and a general observation of how the patient tolerated the procedure. Adverse effects shall be specifically noted and treated promptly.

7. All treatments of whatever nature administered to patients at the institutions maintained by or under the control of the defendants shall accord with the standards of quality and care reasonably expected by and of the medical and psychiatric professions.

8. Any individual having knowledge of any violation with respect to any standard or requirement herein set forth shall bring such matter immediately to the attention of the appropriate Human Rights Committee, the Court or counsel of record in this cause.

9. Any policy, directive or procedure adopted or published by the defendants, or any institution maintained by them or under their control, which is now in effect or which is proposed to take effect in the future and which is inconsistent with the requirements of these standards shall be void and of no effect.

Donaldson v. O'Connor

Kenneth DONALDSON, Plaintiff-Appellee,

v.

J. B. O'CONNOR, M. D. and John Gumanis, M. D., Defendants-Appellants.

No. 73-1843.

United States Court of Appeals, Fifth Circuit.

April 26, 1974.

WISDOM, Circuit Judge:

This case requires us to decide for the first time the far-reaching question whether the Fourteenth Amendment guarantees a right to treatment to persons involuntarily civilly committed to state mental hospitals. The plaintiff-appellee, Kenneth Donaldson, was civilly committed to the Florida State Hospital at Chattahootchee in January 1957, diagnosed as a "paranoid schizophrenic". He remained in that hospital for the next fourteen and a half years. During that time he received little or no psychiatric care or treatment.

Donaldson contends that he had a constitutional right to receive treatment or to be released from the state hospital.

In this action, filed February 24, 1971, he seeks damages under 42 U.S.C. § 1983 [1] against five hospital and state mental health officials who allegedly deprived him of this constitutional right.[2] A jury returned a verdict of $28,500 in compensatory damages, and $10,000 in punitive damages against the two defendants-appellants, Dr. J. B. O'Connor and Dr. John Gumanis. Dr. O'Connor, as Acting Clinical Director of the hospital, was Donaldson's attending physician from the time of his admission until mid-1959. He was Clinical Director of the hospital from mid-1959 until late 1963, and Superintendent thereafter until his retirement February 1, 1971. Dr. John Gumanis was Donaldson's attending physician from the fall of 1959 until the spring of 1967. He was added as a defendant by an amended complaint filed April 20, 1972. The jury returned a verdict in favor of the other three defendants.

Gumanis and O'Connor bring separate appeals to this Court. They challenge the sufficiency of the evidence to support the jury verdict [3] and they contend that the Constitution does not guarantee a right to treatment to mental patients involuntarily civilly committed. Both argue, therefore, that the trial judge erred in denying a motion to dismiss for failure to state a claim and in instructing the jury that civilly committed mental patients have a constitutional right to treatment. In addition, Gumanis raises a number of lesser issues. We hold that the Fourteenth amendment guarantees involuntarily civilly committed mental patients a right to treatment, and that the evidence was sufficient to support the verdict. We also reject the numerous lesser contentions advanced by Gumanis. Accordingly, we affirm the judgment in Donaldson's favor.

I.

To put the legal issues in proper context as well as to discuss the defendants' challenge to the sufficiency of the evidence, it is essential to review the facts in unusual detail.

Donaldson was committed January 3, 1957, on the petition of his father and after a brief hearing before a county judge of Pinellas County, Florida. He was admitted to the Florida State Hospital twelve days later, and soon thereafter was diagnosed as a "paranoid schizophrenic". The committing judge told Donaldson that he was being sent to the hospital for "a few weeks" to "take some of this new medication", after which the judge said that he was certain that Donaldson would be "all right" and would "come back here". Donaldson

---

1. 42 U.S.C. § 1983 provides:

    statute, ordinance, regulation, custom, or usage, of any State or Territory, subjects, or causes to be subjected, any citizen of the United States or other person within the jurisdiction thereof to the deprivation of any rights, privileges, or immunities secured by the Constitution and laws, shall be liable to the party injured in an action at law, suit in equity, or other proper proceeding for redress.

2. Except when the text clearly indicates otherwise, we use the term "defendants" in this opinion to refer to Dr. Gumanis and Dr. O'Connor, against whom judgments were rendered. The other three who were sued were: Dr. Francis G. Walls, who became Acting Superintendent of the Hospital when O'Connor retired from that position in February 1971, and who held that position for about four months; Dr. Milton J. Hirschberg, who became permanent Superintendent,

succeeding O'Connor, in June 1971; and Emmett S. Roberts, Secretary of the Department of Health and Rehabilitative Services in Florida at the time Donaldson filed his First Amended Complaint August 30, 1971.

3. The defendants raised the question of the sufficiency of the evidence on a motion for directed verdict made at the close of the plaintiff's evidence, and renewed at the close of all evidence. The defendants apparently did not move for judgment notwithstanding the verdict after the verdict was returned, but they did move for a new trial. The first ground they asserted in their motion for new trial was that "[t]he verdict is contrary to the clear weight of the evidence, which evidence showed that Defendants reasonably believed in good faith that due to his mental illness and need of treatment Plaintiff was properly confined".

was not released until July 31, 1971, after he had instituted this suit.

There is little dispute about the general nature of the conditions under which Donaldson was confined for almost fifteen years. Donaldson received no commonly accepted psychiatric treatment. Shortly after his first mental examination, Donaldson, a Christian Scientist, refused to take any medication or to submit to electroshock treatments, and he consistently refused to submit to either of these forms of therapy. No other therapy was offered. At trial, Gumanis mentioned "recreational" and "religious" therapy as forms of therapy given Donaldson; but this amounted to allowing Donaldson to attend church and to engage in recreational activities, privileges he probably would have been allowed in a prison. In the oral argument on appeal the appellants' counsel made much of what they called "milieu therapy", which they said was given Donaldson. This was nothing more than keeping Donaldson in a sheltered hospital "milieu" with other mental patients; the defendants did not refer to anything specific about the "milieu" that was in any special way therapeutic.[4] Donaldson was usually confined in a locked room, where, according to his testimony, there were about sixty beds, with little more room between beds than was necessary for a chair; his possessions were kept under the bed. At night he was often awakened by some who had fits and by some "who would torment other patients, screaming and hollering". Then there was "the fear, always the fear you have in your heart, I suppose, when you go to sleep that maybe somebody would jump on you during the night".

A third of the patients in the ward were criminals. Indeed, Donaldson testified, "The entire operation of the ward was geared to criminal patients."[5]

4. "Milieu therapy" is a frequent response by doctors and hospitals to claims by patients that they are receiving inadequate treatment. See Halpern, A Practicing Lawyer Views the Right to Treatment, 1969, 57 Geo.L.J. 782, 786–87, n. 19. Halpern discusses "milieu therapy" in analyzing Rouse v. Cameron, 1966, 125 U.S.App.D.C. 366, 373 F.2d 451, a pioneer case in which the District of Columbia Court of Appeals (Bazelon, J.) held that there was a statutory right to treatment. Halpern notes that "milieu therapy" is an "amorphous and intangible" concept, "the easiest therapeutic claim for an institution to assert and the most difficult for a patient to refute", Halpern, *supra*, at 787 n. 19.

5. Some of Donaldson's testimony relating the conditions under which he lived is worth quoting:
"Q. Now, in the buildings you lived in Department A, were those buildings locked?
A. Yes, sir.
Q. Were the wards you lived on locked?
A. Yes.
Q. Were there metal enclosures on the windows?
A. Yes, padlocks on each window.
Q. Approximately how many beds were there in the rooms where you slept?
A. Sixty some beds.
Q. How close together were they?
A. Some of the beds were touching, the sides touched, and others there was room enough to put a straight chair if we had had a chair.
Q. Did you have chairs in the room you were in?
A. There wasn't a chair in the room I was in. . . .
Q. Now, Mr. Donaldson, you were civilly committed. You had not been charged with any crime, is that right?
A. That is right.
Q. Were there criminal patients on your ward?
A. There were criminal patients on the ward.
Q. Approximately what percent of the population on your ward were criminals?
A. Looking back, roughly, I would say a third. I do not know the figures for the whole department.
Q. Let's just talk about your ward.
A. Okay, I would say about a third in the wards I was in.
Q. Now, did you sleep in the same rooms as the criminal patients?
A. Yes.
Q. Did you get up at the same time?
A. Yes.
Q. Did you eat the same food?
A. Yes.
Q. In the same dining room?
A. Yes.
Q. Did you wear the same clothes?
A. Yes. The entire operation of the wards I was on was geared to the criminal patients.

During his first ten years at the hospital, progress reports on Donaldson's condition were irregularly entered at intervals averaging about one every two and a half months. During those first ten years, he requested grounds privileges and occupational therapy; his requests were denied. In short, he received only the kind of subsistence level custodial care he would have received in a prison, and perhaps less psychiatric treatment than a criminally committed inmate would have received.

At the time Donaldson was admitted to the hospital in 1957, O'Connor was Assistant Clinical Director of the hospital. As Assistant Clinical Director, he was in charge of the hospital's Department A, then the white male ward, where Donaldson was assigned upon his admission to the hospital. In that position, O'Connor was Donaldson's attending physician. At that time, Gumanis was a staff physician in Department A. On July 1, 1959, O'Connor became Clinical Director of the hospital, and in the fall of 1959, Gumanis was placed in charge of Department A, and became Donaldson's attending physician. O'Connor was promoted from the position of Clinical Director to the position of Superintendent July 30, 1963, and served as Superintendent until he retired February 1, 1971. Gumanis served as Donaldson's attending physician until

April 18, 1967, when Donaldson was transferred to Department C, until that time the Negro male ward. After the transfer, Donaldson's attending physician was Dr. Israel Hanenson, the head of Department C until Dr. Hanenson's death in the fall of 1970. After that, until his release, Donaldson's attending physician was Dr. Jesus Rodriguez.

Donaldson brought this suit while he was still a patient at the hospital. In his original complaint, Donaldson sought to bring this suit as a class action on behalf of all patients in the hospital's Department C. In addition to damages, to the plaintiff and to the class, the complaint sought habeas corpus relief directing the release of Donaldson and of the entire class, and sought broad declaratory and injunctive relief requiring the hospital to provide adequate psychiatric treatment.

After Donaldson's release, and after the district court dismissed the action as a class suit, Donaldson, on August 30, 1971, filed his First Amended Complaint. This complaint sought individual damages and renewed Donaldson's prayers for declaratory and injunctive relief to restrain the enforcement of Florida's civil commitment statutes unless Florida provided adequate treatment to its civilly committed mental patients. The complaint asked the district court to convene a three-judge district court to

---

Q. Let me ask you, were you treated any differently from the criminal patients?

A. I was treated worse than the criminal patients.

Q. In what sense were you treated worse?

A. The criminal patients got the attention of the doctors. Generally a doctor makes a report to the court every month.

Q. For the criminal?

A. On the criminal patients, and that would be a pretty heavy case load. It didn't give them time to see the ones who weren't criminal patients.

Q. Was there a place on the ward you had access to for keeping personal possessions?

A. No, not at that time.

Q. What did you do with your personal possessions?

A. I kept mine in a cedar box under the mattress of my bed.

Q. Was there a place in the wards where you could get some privacy?

A. No, not anytime in all of the years I was locked up.

Q. Were you able to get a good nights sleep?

A. No.

Q. Why not?

A. On all of the wards there was the same mixture of patients. There were some patients who had fits during the night. There were some patients who would torment other patients, screaming and hollering, and the fear, always the fear you have in your mind, I suppose, when you go to sleep that maybe somebody will jump on you during the night.

They never did, but you think about those things. It was a lunatic asylum."

consider the plaintiff's attack on the constitutionality of the civil commitment statutes as they then operated. On November 30, however, the plaintiff in a memorandum brief abandoned the prayer that a three-judge court be convened. The prayers for injunctive and declaratory relief therefore were effectively eliminated from the case.

The key allegation in the amended complaint charged that the defendants O'Connor and Walls had "acted in bad faith toward plaintiff and with intentional, malicious, and reckless disregard of his constitutional rights". The complaint alleged examples of such actions, including the denial to Donaldson of grounds privileges; the refusal of the psychiatrists to speak with him, even at his own request; refusal or obstruction of his opportunities for out-of-state discharge, despite a recommendation by a staff conference that he be given such a discharge, and despite the presentation of a signed parental consent to such a discharge. The core of the charge, however, was that Walls and O'Connor acted intentionally and maliciously in "confining Donaldson against his will, knowing that [he] was not physically dangerous to himself or others"; in confining him "knowing that [he] was not receiving adequate treatment, and knowing that absent such treatment the period of his hospitalization would be prolonged"; and that they "intentionally limit[ed] [his] 'treatment' program to 'custodial care' for the greater part of his hospitalization". Corresponding to these allegations, the complaint sought $100,000 damages against Walls and O'Connor.

The trial began November 21, 1972, and continued for four days. The jury returned a verdict awarding Donaldson $17,000 in compensatory damages and $5,000 in punitive damages against O'Connor, and $11,500 in compensatory damages and $5,000 in punitive damages against Gumanis. The jury returned

verdicts in favor of the other three defendants. From the judgment entered on this verdict, Gumanis and O'Connor appeal.

The trial centered, of course, upon the conditions of Donaldson's confinement and upon the defendants' behavior toward Donaldson. On the record as a whole, there was ample evidence to support the jury's reaching any or all of the conclusions set forth in the following subsections in Part I of this opinion.

A. *The defendants unjustifiably withheld from Donaldson specific forms of treatment.*

The evidence establishes that there were at least three forms of treatment the defendants withheld from Donaldson.

First, he was denied grounds privileges. Since the purpose of hospitalization is to restore the capacity for independent community living, one of the most basic modes of treatment is giving a patient an increasing degree of independence and personal responsibility. One of the plaintiff's expert witnesses was Dr. Walter Fox, Director of the Arizona Mental Health Department and former president of the Association of Medical Superintendents of Mental Hospitals. He had interviewed Donaldson and examined his hospital record. Fox testified that confining Donaldson to a locked building, with no opportunity for grounds privileges was not "consistent" with a treatment plan for a patient with Donaldson's history.

Gumanis denied Donaldson a privilege card, even after Donaldson had asked him for one. Fox testified that it would have been "standard psychiatric practice" to extend grounds privileges to a patient of Donaldson's background, condition, and history. Gumanis, in his testimony at trial, could not give a convincing explanation for his refusal of grounds privileges to Donaldson.[6] At

6. Donaldson testified that he had once escaped from the hospital. This occurred around Christmastime 1957, shortly before

the end of the first year Donaldson had spent at Florida State. The hospital records, however, did not show that a fear one point he sought to shift the responsibility for the refusal to O'Connor's shoulders, saying that he recalled having denied privileges after consultation with O'Connor. Later, he testified that at the time in question Donaldson had appeared to him to be "really upset", and that he had "probably" made the decision to deny Donaldson a privilege card on his own. Donaldson testified that soon after his transfer to Department C, Dr. Hanenson, the physician in charge of that department, gave him a privilege card.

The second form of treatment denied Donaldson was occupational therapy. Donaldson testified that Gumanis consistently refused to allow him to enter occupational therapy. This testimony was borne out by a progress note entered in Donaldson's hospital record January 17, 1964. Again, Fox testified that given what he called Donaldson's "social history", Donaldson would have been ideally suited to benefit from occupational therapy. According to Donaldson, Gumanis did not want him to go into occupational therapy, because Gumanis feared that he would learn touch-typing and would use this skill, in Donaldson's words, to "write writs", that is, to prepare habeas corpus petitions. Gumanis gave no reason why he denied Donaldson occupational therapy, although in the course of his testimony he did allude to the fact that he had done so. Not until Donaldson was transferred to Dr. Hanenson's care was he allowed to enter occupational therapy.

Third, the simplest and most routine form of psychiatric treatment is to have a patient talk with a psychiatrist. Donaldson testified that in the eighteen months O'Connor was in direct charge of his case, he spoke with O'Connor "not more than six times", and that the total time he spent talking to O'Connor did not consume more than one hour. He testified that in the eight and one-half years he spent under Gumanis' care, he did not speak with Gumanis more than a total of two hours—an average of about fourteen minutes a year. He testified that neither Gumanis nor O'Connor ever heeded his requests to discuss his case. On one occasion Gumanis said that he "talked only to patients that he wanted to". Gumanis did not recall that conversation. Once again, there was evidence to show that the situation improved when Donaldson was transferred to Dr. Hanenson's care. Donaldson testified that Hanenson managed to speak with him once a week, even though, according to Donaldson, patients were more numerous, psychiatrists fewer, and conditions worse in Hanenson's Department C than they had been in Gumanis's Department A.

B. *The defendants recklessly failed to attend to and treat Donaldson at precisely those junctures when treatment could have most helped Donaldson recover and therefore be released.*

The jury could have concluded that Donaldson should have been marked, at his entrance to the hospital, as a prime candidate for an early release, and that the defendants acted recklessly in failing to treat or attend to him during the early stage of his confinement. Fox testified that, given Donaldson's history,[7] he should have been "pegged" for an "early discharge". Moreover, a progress note entered by Gumanis after his first diagnostic interview with Donaldson, March 25, 1957, recorded that Donaldson "appeared" to be "in remission". Gumanis defined "remission" for the jury as a state "when the patient does not express

---

Donaldson would attempt to escape again motivated the denial of grounds privileges; nor have Gumanis and O'Connor asserted before this Court that such a fear was their reason for denying Donaldson a card.

7. Fourteen years before he was hospitalized in Florida, Donaldson had been hospitalized

at the Marcy State Hospital in New York, with the same diagnosis as that made by the Florida doctors—"paranoid schizophrenic". On that occasion, Donaldson was released after three months.

delusions or paranoid ideas", and told the jury that it was hospital practice to release patients who were in remission. He testified that Donaldson was not released because he wanted to "observe [Donaldson] further". But after that interview the first progress note entered in Donaldson's hospital record is dated four months later; and the next report five months after that. Asked about this, Gumanis first replied, "When you have 900 patients you do that"; later, he insisted that he had seen Donaldson frequently, but had not recorded progress notes after each observation. The jury, however, could have discounted this testimony and concluded that Gumanis acted wantonly in giving a patient who had appeared to be "in remission" the same treatment he gave his 900 other patients.

C. *The defendants wantonly, maliciously, or oppressively blocked efforts by responsible and interested friends and organizations to have Donaldson released to their custody.*

At issue here are two efforts made to secure Donaldson's release, one by Helping Hands, Inc., a Minneapolis organization which runs halfway houses for mental patients and John H. Lembcke, a college friend of Donaldson.

1. *The Helping Hands' attempt to obtain Donaldson's release.*

Helping Hands made an inquiry to the hospital concerning the possibility of releasing Donaldson to its custody by a letter dated June 6, 1963:

> We are interested in the possibility of signing out your patient, Kenneth Donaldson, and taking him as a resident at our halfway house at 3800 Columbus Avenue, Minneapolis. A maximum of six people live here, including our house mother, and myself, as president. At this time we have a room for Kenneth, who has interested us very much through his letters.

Enclosed with the letter was a brochure describing Helping Hands and a letter from the Minneapolis Clinic of Psychiatry and Neurology, stating that "it would be impossible in any of our State Hospitals for a patient to receive the type of attention and care" provided at Helping Hands. The author of this letter pointed out that the woman identified by the letterhead as the founder and director of Helping Hands had "rehabilitated well over a thousand over the years". The letter requested information concerning Donaldson's age, health, and "qualifications for work".

The hospital responded June 17, 1963, in a letter signed by O'Connor, then Clinical Director of the hospital. It gave Donaldson's age, and answered inquiries concerning his health and qualifications for work with the bare statement that Donaldson was "mentally incompetent at the present time". The crisp concluding paragraph read:

> Should he [Donaldson] be released from this Hospital, he will require very strict supervision, which he would not tolerate. Such a release would be to the parents. We see no prospects of his release to any third party at any time in the near future.

The jury could have decided that Gumanis and O'Connor acted wantonly and maliciously in issuing this response, and that this conduct foreclosed an opportunity for Donaldson to win back at least a part of his freedom, and to gain access to a level of psychiatric treatment unavailable to him at the Florida Hospital. Each of the defendants sought to shift the responsibility for sending this curt reply to the other's shoulders. They discussed the question in terms of whether hospital rules, in general, fixed responsibility for deciding whether a patient could be furloughed by the attending physician, or the Superintendent or Clinical Director; they did not discuss it in terms of their recollections of the particular event. The jury would have been justified in finding the two jointly responsible for the incident.

2. *The Lembcke attempt to obtain Donaldson's release.*

John H. Lembcke, a certified public accountant in Binghamton, New York, who is married and has three children, had been a classmate of Donaldson's at Syracuse University in the 1920's. On four occasions, Lembcke sought to have Donaldson released to his custody. The first was on July 3, 1964, when Lembcke informed the hospital that Donaldson was a friend of his, and inquired whether there were "any conditions under which he would be released so that I could bring him back to New York State". The same day the hospital received the letter, O'Connor penciled a note to Gumanis that is attached to the letter in Donaldson's hospital record. The note said:

This man must not be well himself to want to get involved with someone like this patient, who even the recent visiting psychologist considered *dangerous*—Recommend turn it down.

Rich, the new Clinical Director, wrote Lembcke saying that Donaldson had "shown no particular changes mentally", and that if released he would "require complete supervision".

The second inquiry came by letter of November 27, 1964. Again O'Connor appended a note to Gumanis that is in the hospital records. This note gave three reasons for denying Lembcke's request to have Donaldson released to him: parental consent would be required; the patient "would not stay with party mentioned"; and "we don't know anything about party". Gumanis prepared a letter, dated November 27 and again signed by Dr. Rich, "advis-[ing]" Lembcke that Donaldson would "require further hospitalization". The reply did not mention the three reasons for the denial set out in O'Connor's note, and did not request any further information from Lembcke, even though Lembcke in his November 23 letter had offered to provide any information the hospital should request.

The third attempt by Lembcke began with another letter to the hospital, dated December 21, 1965. According to Lembcke's testimony, the hospital responded by saying Donaldson could be released on two conditions: (1) that Lembcke would give Donaldson "adequate supervision" so that the release would not be detrimental to his mental health; and (2) that Lembcke would secure parental permission for Donaldson to go to New York with Lembcke. In May 1966, Lembcke went to Florida, and met with Gumanis and O'Connor. While in Florida he saw Donaldson and obtained from Donaldson's parents a letter dated May 14, 1966, giving their consent to Donaldson's being released to him. Nothing happened. In his testimony Lembcke did not explain how or why he came to abandon this 1966 effort to secure his friend's release.

Lembcke's final and most important effort to secure Donaldson's release began in March 1968. On March 21, the General Staff, at a meeting attended by Gumanis and Hanenson but not by O'Connor, recommended Donaldson's release on a trial visit or out-of-state discharge. On March 24, Lembcke wrote the hospital renewing his offer to take Donaldson. On March 28, the hospital responded, imposing three conditions on Donaldson's release: (1) that Lembcke be willing to come for Donaldson; (2) that he be willing to supervise Donaldson; and (3) that he be willing to take Donaldson to a psychiatrist if Donaldson needed treatment. By letter of March 31, Lembcke acceded to these conditions. On April 4, the hospital replied with a letter imposing two additional conditions: (1) a detailed statement concerning the home supervision Donaldson would be given; and (2) written authorization for the release from Donaldson's parents. Lembcke wrote back giving the hospital the information about home supervision it had requested. The hospital replied by again saying it would be necessary to obtain the written consent of Donaldson's parents.

On September 18, 1968, Lembcke wrote the hospital, enclosing a photocopy of the notarized written permission Donaldson's parents had signed May 14, 1966. The hospital responded in a letter dated September 24, signed by Dr. Rich. The letter informed Lembcke that Donaldson had been mentally ill for many years, that he "still express[ed] delusional thinking" and that "it would not be fair to you or to him to release him from the hospital at this time without adequate planning". The letter added, in its final paragraph, that it would be necessary for the hospital to have more recent authorization from Donaldson's nearest relative than the one Lembcke had proffered. At that point, Lembcke gave up; whenever he met the conditions imposed by the hospital officials, new conditions were imposed. As he put it, "after requirements were met, requirements were increased".

One other facet of Lembcke's last attempt to secure Donaldson's release bears mention. As noted, O'Connor did not attend the Staff Conference which had recommended Donaldson's release March 21. O'Connor first learned of the hospital's recommendation in June, when Donaldson wrote to the Division Director of the hospital concerning the effort being made to release him. The division director forwarded the letter to O'Connor, who in turn forwarded it to Hanenson, asking for information concerning the proposed release. Hanenson responded with a memorandum dated June 17. Across the bottom of this memorandum, O'Connor pencilled in the remark, "the record will show, I believe, we have been through this before and decided Mr. Lembcke would not properly supervise the patient". It was not clear when O'Connor supposed this "decision" to have been made, and in his deposition O'Connor was unable to locate any record of it in the hospital record. Moreover, there were suggestions in the record that Dr. O'Connor's conduct, in this and other respects, was influenced by his knowledge of Donaldson's history

of writing letters to the press and to outside officials. From all of this evidence, the jury would have been justified in concluding that the frustration of Lembcke's effort to secure Donaldson's release in 1968 was entirely or primarily the result of O'Connor's bad faith intervention or, at the least, that the intervention was in reckless disregard of Donaldson's rights.

D. *The defendants continued to confine Donaldson knowing he was not dangerous, or with reckless disregard for whether he was dangerous.*

Three of the plaintiff's expert witnesses—Fox, Raymond D. Fowler, Jr., Chairman of the Psychology Department at the University of Alabama and former President of both the Alabama and Southern Psychological Associations, and Julian Davis, Director of the Psychology Department at the Florida State Hospital—testified that they did not believe Donaldson was dangerous. Fox's and Fowler's opinions were based upon the hospital records, Donaldson's pyschological reports, Donaldson's past history, and raw data from his physchological examinations. Lembcke testified that in his half century of having known Donaldson, he had never known Donaldson to be "violent", "aggressive", or "belligerent"; that, on the contrary, he knew Donaldson to be a "gentle" man. Dr. Walls testified that he did not believe Donaldson was physically dangerous; Gumanis himself conceded that he did not think Donaldson dangerous while Donaldson was in the hospital, although he said he could not predict what Donaldson would be like outside the hospital. There was no evidence in the record of Donaldson's ever having been violent in any way.

On the basis of this testimony the jury would have been justified in finding that Donaldson was non-dangerous, and in inferring that the defendants knew him to be so.

E. *The defendants did not do the best they could with available resources.*

As they did in the district court, the defendants on appeal pitch their defense in substantial part on their contention that they did the best they could with limited resources available to the state psychiatric hospital. Donaldson rebuts this contention, first, by pointing out the contrast between the treatment he received from the defendants and that he received from Hanenson. Hanenson allowed him grounds privileges and occupational therapy, spoke with him frequently, and within a year of taking charge of his case arranged a staff conference that recommended his release. Second, he relies on the testimony of Fox and the other experts to the effect that Gumanis and O'Connor failed to take steps that would have been open to them to take, even given the admittedly stark limitations on the resources available to them. We agree that these two considerations were a sufficient basis for the jury to reject the defendants' defense that they did the best they could with available resources.

We turn now to the novel and important question whether civilly committed mental patients have a constitutional right to treatment.

II.

[1]   The theory of Donaldson's cause of action under section 1983 was set forth in three of the instructions given by the trial judge. The first, instruction number 34, was a variation of a standard form "boiler plate" instruction found in 2 Dewitt & Blackmer's Federal Jury Practice & Instructions, 1970, § 87.05 (2d ed.) This instruction stated that there were four basic elements Don-

aldson had to prove to make out a claim under § 1983: (1) that the defendants "confined plaintiff against his will, knowing that he was not mentally ill or dangerous, and knowing that if mentally ill he was not receiving treatment for his mental illness"; (2) that defendants "then and there acted under the color of state law"; (3) that defendants' "acts and conduct deprived the plaintiff of his federal constitutional right not to be denied his liberty without due process of law as that phrase is defined and explained in these instructions"; and (4) that the defendants' "acts and conduct were the proximate cause of injury and consequent damage to the plaintiff". The other two instructions, 37 and 38, were the relevant instructions "defin[ing] and explain[ing]" the "phrase", "federal constitutional right not to be denied or deprived of his liberty without due process of law", within the meaning of instruction 34. These instructions told the jury:

37.   You are instructed that a person who is involuntarily civilly committed to a mental hospital does have a constitutional right to receive such individual treatment as will give him a realistic opportunity to be cured or to improve his mental condition.

38.   The purpose of involuntary hospitalization is treatment and not mere custodial care or punishment if a patient is not dangerous to himself or others. Without such treatment there is no justification, from a constitutional standpoint, for continued confinement.

The propriety of these two instructions is the heart of the question raised by both O'Connor and Gumanis in their appeals.[8]

---

8.   As a threshhold matter, Donaldson suggests that the objections to these instructions are not properly before this Court. He notes that the defendants did not object to that instruction either when the proposed instructions were discussed in chambers, or after the charge was read to the jury. The

defendants did, however, object to what were then the plaintiff's proposed instructions 37 and 38 in a pretrial brief filed before the Court. There they asked that those instructions be replaced with an instruction that "[y]ou are instructed that a person who is committed to a mental hospital has a right

[2] The question for decision, whether patients involuntarily civilly committed in state mental hospitals have a constitutional right to treatment, has never been addressed by any of the federal courts of appeals. Four district courts, however, have decided the question within the last three years, three of which held that there is a constitutional right to treatment.[9] The Court of Appeals for the District of Columbia Circuit, in a landmark case decided eight years ago, took note in dictum of the existence and seriousness of the question, although in the same case the court held that the Hospitalization of the Mentally Ill Act of 1964 [10] creates a *statutory* right to treatment on the part of mental patients in the District of Columbia.[11] The idea of a constitutional right to treatment has received an unusual amount of scholarly discussion and support,[12] and there is now an enormous range of precedent relevant to, although

to be released through judicial process when through no fault of his own treatment is not afforded and he is not dangerous to society or to himself". The trial judge refused this request, and gave the two instructions as the plaintiffs had proposed them. It is settled that "a failure to object may be disregarded if a party's position has previously been made clear to the court and it is plain that a further objection would be unavailing". 9 C. Wright & A. Miller, Federal Practice & Procedure § 2553 at 639–40; see, e. g., Mays v. Dealers Transit, 7 Cir. 1971, 441 F.2d 1344; Steinhauser v. Hertz Corp., 2 Cir. 1970, 421 F.2d 1169. We find that was the case here, and therefore we consider that the objections are properly before the Court.

9. Two cases hold that there is a right to treatment for civilly committed mentally ill patients. Wyatt v. Stickney, M.D.Ala.1971, 325 F.Supp. 781, *on submission of proposed standards by defendants,* 334 F.Supp. 1341, enforced, 1972, 344 F.Supp. 373, 387, appeal docketed sub nom., Wyatt v. Aderholt, No. 72–2634, 5 Cir. Aug. 1, 1972; Stachulak v. Coughlin, N.D.Ill., 1973, 364 F.Supp. 686. One has held civilly committed mentally ill patients enjoy no right to treatment. Burnham v. Department of Public Health, N.D. Ga.1972, 349 F.Supp. 1335, appeal docketed, No. 72–3110, 5 Cir. Oct. 4, 1972.

A fourth case has recently held that civilly committed mentally retarded patients have a right to treatment. Welsch v. Likins, No. 4–72–Civ. 451, D.Minn. Feb. 15, 1974, 373 F.Supp. 487.

10. D.C.Code Ann. § 21–501.

11. Rouse v. Cameron, 1966, 125 U.S.App.D. C. 366, 373 F.2d 451. Chief Judge Bazelon wrote for the Court:

Absence of treatment "might draw into question 'the constitutionality of [this] mandatory commitment section' as applied." (1) Lack of improvement raises a question of procedural due process where the commitment is under D.C.Code § 24–301 rath-

er than under the civil commitment statute, for under § 24–301 commitment is summary, in contrast with civil commitment safeguards. It does not rest on any finding of present insanity and dangerousness but, on the contrary, on a jury's reasonable doubt that the defendant was sane when he committed the act charged. Commitment on this basis is permissible because of its humane therapeutic goals. (2) Had appellant been found criminally responsible, he could have been confined a year, at most, however dangerous he might have been. He has been confined four years and the end is not in sight. Since this difference rests only on need for treatment, a failure to supply treatment may raise a question of due process of law. It has also been suggested that a failure to supply treatment may violate the equal protection clause. (3) Indefinite commitment without treatment of one who has been found not criminally responsible may be so inhumane as to be "cruel and unusual punishment." [Footnotes and citations omitted]

Id. at 453.

12. The seminal article in the field is Birnbaum, The Right to Treatment, 1960, 46 A. B.A. Journal 499. Much of the commentary in the area was stimulated by the *Rouse* decision. *E. g.,* Symposium—The Right to Treatment, 1969, 57 Geo.L.J. 673 (11 articles, 218 pages); Bazelon, Implementing the Right to Treatment, 1969, 36 U.Chi.L.Rev. 742; Birnbaum, Some Remarks on "The Right to Treatment," 1971, 23 Ala.L.Rev. 623; Chambers, Alternatives to Civil Commitment of the Mentally Ill: Practical Guides and Constitutional Imperatives, 1969, 70 Mich.L.Rev. 1108; Katz, The Right to Treatment—An Enchanting Legal Fiction? 1969, U.Chi.L.Rev. 755; Drake, Enforcing the Right to Treatment: Wyatt v. Stickney, 1972, 10 Am.Crim.L.Rev. 587; Morris, "Criminality" and the Right to Treatment, 1969, U.Chi.L.Rev. 784; Note, The Nascent Right to Treatment, 1967, 53 Va.L.Rev.

not squarely in point with, the issue.[13] The idea has been current at least since 1960, since the publication in the May 1960 issue of the American Bar Association Journal of an article by Dr. Morton Birnbaum, a forensic medical doctor now generally credited with being the father of the idea of a right to treatment.[14] The A.B.A. Journal editorially endorsed the idea shortly after the publication of Dr. Birnbaum's article.[15]

We hold that a person involuntarily civilly committed to a state mental hospital has a constitutional right to receive such individual treatment as will give him a reasonable opportunity to be cured or to improve his mental condition.

In reaching this result, we begin by noting the indisputable fact that civil commitment entails a "massive curtailment of liberty" in the constitutional sense. Humphrey v. Cady, 1972, 405 U.S. 504, 509, 92 S.Ct. 1048, 31 L.Ed.2d 394. The destruction of an individual's personal freedoms effected by civil commitment is scarcely less total than that effected by confinement in a penitentiary. Indeed, civil commitment, because it is for an indefinite term, may in some ways involve a more serious abridgement of personal freedom than imprisonment for commission of a crime usually does. Civil commitment involves stigmatizing the affected individuals, and the stigma attached, though in theory less severe than the stigma attached to criminal conviction, may in reality be as severe, or more so.[16] Since civil com-

mitment involves deprivations of liberty of the kind with which the due process clause is frequently concerned, that clause has the major role in regulating government actions in this area.

Beyond this, the conclusion that the due process clause guarantees a right to treatment rests upon a two-part theory. The first part begins with the fundamental, and all but universally accepted, proposition that "any nontrivial governmental abridgement of [any] freedom [which is part of the 'liberty' the Fourteenth Amendment says shall not be denied without due process of law] must be justified in terms of some 'permissible governmental goal.'" Tribe, Foreward—Toward a Model of Roles in the Due Process of Life and Law, 86 Harv. L.Rev. 1, 17 (1973). Once this "fairly sweeping concept of substantive due process" is assumed, *id.* at 5 n. 26,[17] the next step is to ask precisely what government interests justify the massive abridgement of liberty civil commitment entails. Typically, three distinct grounds for civil commitment are recognized by state statutes: danger to self; danger to others; and need for treatment, or for "care", "custody", or "supervision". Jackson v. Indiana, 1972, 406 U.S. 715, 737, 92 S.Ct. 1845, 32 L. Ed.2d 435; see Note, Civil Commitment of the Mentally Ill: Theories and Procedures, 1966, 79 Harv.L.Rev. 1288, 1289–97; Note, The Nascent Right to Treatment, 1967, 53 Va.L.Rev. 1134, 1138–39.[18] It is analytically useful to conceive

---

1134; Note, Civil Restraint, Mental Illness, and the Right to Treatment, 1967, 77 Yale L.J. 87; 80 Harv.L.Rev. 898 (1967).

13. See cases cited at nn. 23–44 *infra.*

14. Birnbaum, The Right to Treatment, 1960, 46 A.B.A.J. 499.

15. Editorial, A New Right, 1960, 46 A.B.A.J. 516.

16. On the recognition that stigmatization constitutes a deprivation of liberty in the constitutional sense, see Board of Regents v. Roth, 1972, 408 U.S. 564, 573, 92 S.Ct. 2701, 33 L.Ed.2d 548, 558–559.

17. *See also* Ely, The Wages of Crying Wolf: A Comment on Roe v. Wade, 1973, 82 Yale L.J. 920, 935 & n. 91; Roe v. Wade, 1973, 410 U.S. 113, 172–173, 93 S.Ct. 705, 35 L. Ed.2d 147 (Rehnquist, J., dissenting); Doe v. Bolton, 1973, 410 U.S. 179, 223, 93 S.Ct. 739, 35 L.Ed.2d 201 (White, J., dissenting).

18. In *Jackson,* the Supreme Court, relying upon an American Bar Foundation study, found that in nine states the sole criterion for involuntary commitment was the danger to self or others; that in 18 other states the patient's need for care or treatment was an alternative basis; that the need for care

of these grounds as falling into two categories, one consisting of a "police power" rationales for confinement, the other of a *"parens patriae"* rationales.[19] Danger to others is a "police power" rationale; need for care or treatment a *"parens patriae"* rationale. Danger to self combines elements of both.

The key point of the first part of the theory of a due process right to treatment is that where, as in Donaldson's case, the rationale for confinement is the *"parens patriae"* rationale that the patient is in need of treatment, the due process clause requires that minimally adequate treatment be in fact provided. This in turn requires that, at least for the nondangerous patient, constitutionally minimum standards of treatment be established and enforced. As Judge Johnson expressed it in the *Wyatt* case: "To deprive any citizen of his or her liberty upon the altruistic theory that the confinement is for humane therapeutic reasons and then fail to provide adequate treatment violates the very fundamentals of due process." Wyatt v. Stickney, *supra*, 325 F.Supp. at 785. Or as Justice Cutter, speaking for the Supreme Judicial Court of Massachusetts, put it: "Convinement of mentally ill persons, not found guilty of crime, without affording them reasonable treatment also raises serious questions of deprivation of liberty without due process of law. As we said in the *Page* case [citation omitted], of a statute permitting

comparable confinement, 'to be sustained as a nonpenal statute . . . it is necessary that the remedial aspect of confinement . . . have foundation in fact.' " Nason v. Superintendent, Bridgewater Hospital, 1968, 353 Mass. 604, 612, 233 N.E.2d 908, 913. This key step in the theory also draws considerable support from, if indeed it is not compelled by, the Supreme Court's recent decision in Jackson v. Indiana, 1972, 406 U.S. 715, 92 S.Ct. 1845, 32 L.Ed.2d 435. In *Jackson,* the Supreme Court established the rule that "[a]t the least, due process requires that the nature and duration of commitment bear some reasonable relation to the purposes for which the individual is committed". 406 U.S. at 738.[20] If the "purpose" of commitment is treatment, and treatment is not provided, then the "nature" of the commitment bears no "reasonable relation" to its "purpose", and the constitutional rule of *Jackson* is violated.

[3, 4] This much represents the first part of the theory of a due process right to treatment; persons committed under what we have termed a *parens patriae* ground for commitment must be given treatment lest the involuntary commitment amount to an arbitrary exercise of government power proscribed by the due process clause. The second part of the theory draws no distinctions between persons committed under *"parens patriae"* rationales and those committed under "police power" rationales. This

---

or treatment was the sole basis in six other states; and a few states had no statutory criteria at all and "presumably le[ft] the determination to judicial discretion". 406 U.S. at 737 n. 19, citing American Bar Foundation, The Mentally Disabled and the Law (rev.ed.1971) at 36–49.

19. See Note, The Nascent Right to Treatment, 1967, 53 Va.L.Rev. 1134, 1138–39.

20. *Jackson* involved a mentally defective deaf mute who was committed after the court determined that he was incompetent to stand trial. Since the mental and physical defects which were the cause of his inability were not susceptible to treatment and not likely to improve during his confinement, it was

unlikely that he would ever become competent to stand trial. In the circumstances, the Supreme Court held that its rule that "the nature and duration of commitment bear some reasonable relation to the purpose for which the individual is committed" permitted the state to confine Jackson under the provisions for the commitment of those found incompetent to stand trial only for "the reasonable period of time necessary to determine whether there is a substantial probability that he will attain that capacity [to stand trial] in the foreseeable future". It held further that even if it were determined that he was likely to become able to stand trial, "his continued commitment [would have to be] justified by progress toward that goal". 406 U.S. at 738.

part begins with the recognition that, under our system of justice, long-term detention is, as a matter of due process, generally permitted only when an individual is (1) proved, in a proceeding subject to the rigorous constitutional limitations of the due process clause of the fourteenth amendment and the Bill of Rights, (2) to have committed a *specific act* defined as an offense against the state. See Powell v. Texas, 1968, 392 U.S. 514, 533, 542–543, 88 S.Ct. 2145, 20 L.Ed.2d 1254 (Black, J., concurring). Moreover, detention, under the criminal process, is usually allowed only for a period of time explicitly fixed by the prisoner's sentence. The second part of the theory of a due process right to treatment is based on the principle that when the three central limitations on the government's power to detain— that detention be in retribution for a specific offense; that it be limited to a fixed term; and that it be permitted after a proceeding where fundamental

procedural safeguards are observed—are absent, there must be a *quid pro quo* extended by the government to justify confinement.[21] And the *quid pro quo* most commonly recognized is the provision of rehabilitative treatment, or, where rehabilitation is impossible, minimally adequate habilitation and care, beyond the subsistence level custodial care that would be provided in a penitentiary.[22]

This second part of the theory draws a wide range of support from a variety of precedents. The relevant cases have arisen in five major procedural contexts.

The earliest group of relevant cases consists of cases decided on habeas corpus petitions brought by citizens held under provisions for various kinds of "nonpenal" confinement, who were being held in correctional facilities for prisoners convicted of crimes. These cases uniformly held that, where detention is "nonpenal" in theory, the very least that

---

21. In Welsch v. Likins, 1974, 373 F.Supp. 487, the District of Minnesota described, and rejected, a different *quid pro quo* rationale for a right to treatment. We also reject the rationale described by the *Welsch* court, and the rationale we embrace should be carefully contrasted with it:

> One theory is that commitment pursuant to civil statutes generally lacks the procedural safeguards afforded those charged with criminal offense. The constitutional justification for this abridgment of *procedural rights* is that the purpose of commitment is treatment. (Emphasis supplied).

Welsch v. Likins, 373 F.Supp. at 496. *See also* Inmates of Boys' Training School v. Affleck, D.R.I.1972, 346 F.Supp. 1354, 1368; Rouse v. Cameron, 1966, 125 U.S.App.D.C. 366, 373 F.2d 451, 453 (Bazelon, C. J.); Note, Civil Restraint, Mental Illness, and the Right to Treatment, 1967, 77 Yale L.J. 87, 90–91, 102–03 & nn. 62–63.

22. Adequate and effective treatment is constitutionally required because, absent treatment, the hospital is transformed "into a penitentiary where one could be held indefinitely for no convicted offense." Wyatt v. Stickney, M.D.Ala.1971, 325 F.Supp. 781, 784, quoting Ragsdale v. Overholser,

1960, 108 U.S.App.D.C. 308, 281 F.2d 943, 950 (Fahy, J., concurring).

Of the various formulations of this "*quid pro quo*" theory we have found, perhaps the most successful is that made by Professor Nicholas Kittrie, writing specifically about confinement of juveniles, but articulating a theory equally applicable to civil commitment of mentally ill persons:

> Our society has increasingly divested certain groups from the traditional criminal justice court and, acting under its asserted role of *parens patriae*, substituted new therapeutic controls.
>
> *   *   *   *   *
>
> A new concept of substantive due process is evolving in [this] therapeutic realm. This concept is founded upon a recognition of the concurrency between the state's exercise of sanctioning powers and its assumption of the duties of social responsibility. Its implication is that effective treatment must be the *quid pro quo* for society's right to exercise its *parens patriae* controls. Whether specifically recognized by statutory enactment or implicitly derived from the constitutional requirements of due process, the right to treatment exists.

Kittrie, Can the Right to Treatment Remedy the Ills of the Juvenile Process? 1969, 57 Geo.L.J. at 851–52, 870.

is required is that the persons be confined in a facility other than a prison.[23]

Later cases expand the view of these cases by holding not only that persons held under provisions for "nonpenal" confinement be held elsewhere than in a prison, but that they must be held in places where the conditions are *actually* therapeutic.[24]

The third line of relevant cases are those where the constitutionality of various modern "nonpenal" statutes—notably sex-offender and defective-delinquent statutes—provide for the confinement of habitual criminal offenders to protect society and to provide rehabilitative care. The decisions have upheld such statutes, but the courts have usually added the proviso that the constitutionality of the statute is conditioned upon the *realization* of the statutory promise of rehabilitative treatment.[25]

The fourth set of cases, highlighted by Rouse v. Cameron[26] and Nason v. Superintendent of Bridgewater State Hospital,[27] consists of cases where individuals under confinement have brought habeas corpus petitions challenging their confinement on the ground that they were not receiving treatment. This is a diverse group of cases; in most of them, the challenge to confinement for lack of treatment has been combined with challenges brought on other grounds, and often the other grounds are the subject of the decisions. Among these cases, however, we have found none where any court has declared that no right to treatment exists, and we have found none explicitly recognizing a *constitutional* right to treatment. When they hold that there is a right to treatment, the cases usually either rest on statutory grounds, or are ambiguous as to whether they are resting upon statutory or con-

---

23. Benton v. Reid, 1956, 98 U.S.App.D.C. 27, 231 F.2d 780; Commonwealth v. Page, 1958, 339 Mass. 313, 159 N.E.2d 82; In re Maddox, 1958, 351 Mich. 358, 88 N.W.2d 470; *cf.* Miller v. Overholser, 1953, 92 U.S.App. D.C. 110, 206 F.2d 415.

24. But this mandatory commitment provision rests upon a supposition, namely, the necessity for treatment of the mental condition which led to the acquittal by reason of insanity. And this necessity for treatment presupposes in turn that treatment will be accorded.
Ragsdale v. Overholser, 1960, 108 U.S.App.D. C. 308, 281 F.2d 943, 950 (Fahy, J., concurring), quoted with approval, Darnell v. Cameron, 1965, 121 U.S.App.D.C. 58, 348 F.2d 64, 67–68, (Bazelon, C. J.) ; Sas v. Maryland, 4 Cir. 1964, 334 F.2d 506, 517, cert. dismissed as improvidently granted sub nom., Murel v. Baltimore City Crim.Ct., 1972, 407 U.S. 355, 92 S.Ct. 2091, 32 L.Ed.2d 791; Commonwealth v. Page, 1959, 339 Mass. 313, 317, 159 N.E.2d 82, 85.

25. For those in the category [of defective delinquents] it [the defective delinquents statute] would substitute psychiatric treatment for punishment in the conventional sense and would free them from confinement, not when they have "paid their debt to society," but when they have been sufficiently cured to make it reasonably safe to release them. With this humanitarian and progressive approach to the problem no person who has deplored

the inadequacies of conventional penological practices can complain. But a statute though "fair on its face and impartial in appearance" may be fraught with the possibility of abuse in that if not administered in the spirit in which it is conceived it can become a mere device for warehousing the obnoxious and antisocial elements of society. . . . *Deficiencies in staff, facilities, and finances would undermine the efficacy of the Institution and the justification for the law, and ultimately the constitutionality of its application.* [Footnotes omitted]
Sas v. Maryland, 4 Cir. 1964, 334 F.2d 506, 517, cert. dismissed as improvidently granted sub nom. Murel v. Baltimore City Crim.Ct. 1972, 407 U.S. 355, 92 S.Ct. 2091, 32 L.Ed. 2d 791 (emphasis supplied).
See also Davy v. Sullivan, M.D.Ala.1973, 354 F.Supp. 1320 (sex offender statute) (three-judge court)

26. 1966, 125 U.S.App.D.C. 366, 373 F.2d 451 (Bazelon, C. J.). The District of Columbia Circuit has reaffirmed its *Rouse* holding on numerous occasions. See, *e. g.,* In re Curry, 1971, 147 U.S.App.D.C. 28, 452 F.2d 1360; Covington v. Harris, 1969, 136 U.S.App.D.C. 35, 419 F.2d 617; Tribby v. Cameron, 1967, 126 U.S.App.D.C. 327, 379 F.2d 104; Dobson v. Cameron, 127 U.S.App.D.C. 324, 383 F.2d 519; Millard v. Cameron, 1966, 125 U. S.App.D.C. 383, 373 F.2d 468.

27. 353 Mass. 604, 233 N.E.2d 908 (1968) (Cutter, J.).

stitutional grounds.[28] But in all cases, the courts have at least sustained the right of a petitioner to a hearing to develop the facts supporting his claim that he is not receiving treatment.[29]

Fifth, and last, among the groups of cases is the spate of recent cases brought as class actions in federal court, seeking broad forms of injunctive and declaratory relief requiring that adequate treatment be provided in state-run facilities. The cases have included attacks on conditions in many types of facilities—including facilities for the mentally ill,[30] the mentally retarded,[31] juvenile delinquents [32] or nondelinquent ju-

veniles held as being "persons in need of supervision".[33]

Taken together, these five sets of cases constitute a near unanimous recognition that governments must afford a *quid pro quo* when they confine citizens in circumstances where the conventional limitations of the criminal process are inapplicable. These five groups include cases decided by all levels of courts—the Supreme Court,[34] the courts of appeals,[35] the federal district courts,[36] and the state courts.[37] One or another of them concerns each of the major forms of "nonpenal confinement: from those with a heavy police power emphasis, such as confinement of sex offenders [38]

28. *But see* Stachulak v. Coughlin, N.D.Ill. 1973, 364 F.Supp. 686, a case of this kind, citing *Wyatt* and holding there is a constitutional right to treatment.

29. *E. g.*, Humphrey v. Cady, 1972, 405 U.S. 504, 92 S.Ct. 1048, 31 L.Ed.2d 394 (characterizing committed sex offender's claim that he was not receiving treatment a "substantial constitutional claim", and remanding for a hearing on, inter alia, that issue).

30. See cases cited in note 9 *supra*.

31. Wyatt v. Stickney, M.D.Ala.1972, 344 F. Supp. 387; Welsch v. Likins, D.Minn.1974, 373 F.Supp. 487. *Contra*, New York State Ass'n for Retarded Children, Inc. v. Rockefeller, E.D.N.Y.1973, 357 F.Supp. 752.

32. Nelson v. Heyne, 7 Cir. 1974, 491 F.2d 352, aff'g N.D.Ind.1972, 355 F.Supp. 451; Inmates of Boys' Training School v. Affleck, D.R.I.1972, 346 F.Supp. 1354; Morales v. Turman, E.D.Tex.1973, 364 F.Supp. 166.

33. Martarella v. Kelley, S.D.N.Y.1972, 349 F.Supp. 575, enforced, 359 F.Supp. 478.
   The closest the Supreme Court has come to speaking directly on the second, more important part of the due process right to treatment theory we articulate, came in In re Gault, 1967, 387 U.S. 1, 22 n. 30, 87 S.Ct. 1428, 18 L.Ed.2d 527, in which the Court, discussing the context of juvenile confinement, wrote:
   While we are concerned only with procedure before the juvenile court in this case, it should be noted that to the extent that the special procedures for juveniles are thought to be justified by the special consideration and treatment afforded them,

   there is reason to doubt that juveniles always receive the benefits of such a *quid pro quo* . . . The high rate of juvenile recidivism casts some doubt upon the adequacy of treatment afforded juveniles . . .

   In fact some courts have recently indicated that appropriate treatment is essential to the validity of juvenile custody, and therefore that a juvenile may challenge the validity of his custody on the ground that he is not in fact receiving any special treatment.

34. Jackson v. Indiana, 1972, 406 U.S. 715, 92 S.Ct. 1845, 32 L.Ed.2d 435; Humphrey v. Cady, 1972, 405 U.S. 504, 92 S.Ct. 1048, 31 L.Ed.2d 394; McNeil v. Director, Patuxent Institution, 1972, 407 U.S. 245, 92 S.Ct. 2083, 32 L.Ed.2d 719.

35. *E. g.*, Nelson v. Heyne, *supra* note 39; Sas v. Maryland, 4 Cir. 1964, 334 F.2d 506, cert. dismissed as improvidently granted sub nom., Murel v. Baltimore City Crim.Ct., 1972, 407 U.S. 355, 92 S.Ct. 2091, 32 L.Ed. 2d 791; Rouse v. Cameron, 1966, 125 U.S. App.D.C. 366, 373 F.2d 541.

36. *E. g.*, cases cited in nn. 9, 31–33, *supra*.

37. *E. g.*, Nason v. Superintendent, Bridgewater Hospital, 1968, 353 Mass. 604, 233 N.E. 2d 908; Commonwealth v. Page, 1959, 339 Mass. 313, 159 N.E.2d 82; In re Maddox, 1958, 351 Mich. 358, 88 N.W.2d 470.

38. *E. g.*, Humphrey v. Cady, 1972, 405 U.S. 504, 92 S.Ct. 1048, 31 L.Ed.2d 394; Davy v. Sullivan, M.D.Ala.1973, 354 F.Supp. 1320 (three-judge court); Commonwealth v. Page, 1959, 339 Mass. 313, 159 N.E.2d 82.

or defective delinquents,[39] of persons acquitted by reason of insanity,[40] or of persons held incompetent to stand trial;[41] those with a heavy *parens patriae* emphasis, such as confinement of the mentally retarded,[42] or of juveniles;[43] and those—such as civil commitment of the mentally ill[44]—with elements of both rationales behind them.

The appellants argue strenuously that a right to constitutionally adequate treatment should not be recognized, because such a right cannot be governed by judicially manageable or ascertainable standards. In making the argument, they rely heavily upon the Northern District of Georgia's decision in Burnham v. Department of Public Health, 1972, 349 F.Supp. 1335, 1341–1343. In *Burnham*, the district judge held that a class action seeking declaratory and injunctive relief requiring the Georgia Department of Public Health to provide treatment at Georgia mental hospitals presented a nonjusticiable controversy. He quoted Baker v. Carr, 1962, 369 U.S. 186, 198, 82 S.Ct. 691, 700, 7 L.Ed.2d

663, for the proposition that determining whether a suit was justiciable requires determining whether "the duty asserted can be judicially identified and its breach judicially determined, and whether protection for the right asserted can be judicially molded". 349 F. Supp. at 1341, quoting 369 U.S. at 198. He then cited the ambiguity of the dictionary definition of treatment, a passage from a law review article noting the fact that there are as many as forty different methods of psychotherapy,[45] and a passage from the Supreme Court's decision in Greenwood v. United States, 1956, 350 U.S. 366, 76 S.Ct. 410, 100 L. Ed. 412, concerning the "tentativeness" and "uncertainty" of "professional judgment" in the mental health field.[46] He concluded: "[T]he claimed duty (i. e. to 'adequately' or 'constitutionally treat') defies judicial identity and therefore prohibits its breach from being judicially defined." 349 F.Supp. at 1342.

The defendants' argument can be answered on two levels. First, we doubt whether, even if we were to concede that

39. *E. g.*, Sas v. Maryland, 4 Cir. 1964, 334 F.2d 506, cert. dismissed as improvidently granted sub nom., Murel v. Baltimore City Crim.Ct., 407 U.S. 355, 92 S.Ct. 2091, 32 L. Ed.2d 791.

40. *E. g.*, Rouse v. Cameron, 1966, 125 U.S. App.D.C. 366, 373 F.2d 451 (Bazelon, C. J.); Darnell v. Cameron, 1965, 121 U.S.App. D.C. 58, 348 F.2d 64 (Bazelon, C. J.); Ragsdale v. Overholser, 1960, 108 U.S.App. D.C. 308, 281 F.2d 943 (Burger, J.).

41. Jackson v. Indiana, 1972, 406 U.S. 715, 92 S.Ct. 1845, 32 L.Ed.2d 435. *See also* Greenwood v. United States, 1956, 350 U.S. 366, 76 S.Ct. 410, 100 L.Ed. 412; United States v. Pardue, D.Conn.1973, 354 F.Supp. 1377; United States v. Jackson, N.D.Cal.1969, 306 F.Supp. 4.

42. *E. g.*, Wyatt v. Stickney, M.D.Ala.1972, 344 F.Supp. 387; Welsch v. Likins, No. 4–72–Civ. 451, D.Minn. Feb. 15, 1974, noted, 42 U.S.L.W. 1141–42.

43. Cases cited in notes 32–33.

44. Cases cited in note 9 *supra.*

45. Levine [M. Levine, Psychotherapy in Medical Practice] lists 40 methods of psychotherapy. Among these, he includes physical treatment, medicinal treatment, reas-

surance, authoritative firmness, hospitalization, ignoring of certain symptoms and attitudes, satisfaction of neurotic needs and bibliotherapy. In addition, there are physical methods of psychiatric therapy, such as the prescription of sedatives and tranquilizers, the induction of convulsions by drugs and electricity, and brain surgery. *Obviously, the term "psychiatric treatment" covers everything that may be done under medical auspices—and more.* If mental treatment is all the things Levine and others tell us it is, how are we to determine whether or not patients in mental hospitals receive adequate amounts of it?
Szasz, The Right to Psychiatric Treatment: Rhetoric and Reality, 1969, 57 Geo.L.J. 740, 741.

46. . . . [T]heir [two court-appointed psychiatrists] testimony illustrates the uncertainty of diagnosis in this field and the tentativeness of professional judgment. The only certain thing that can be said about the present state of knowledge and therapy regarding mental disease is that science has not reached finality of judgment.
Greenwood v. United States, 1956, 350 U.S. 366, 375, 76 S.Ct. 410, 415, 100 L.Ed. 412.

courts are incapable of formulating standards of adequate treatment in the abstract, we could or should for that reason alone hold that no right to treatment can be recognized or enforced. There will be cases—and the case at bar is one—where it will be possible to make determination whether a given individual has been denied his right to treatment without formulating in the abstract what constitutes "adequate" treatment. In this case, the jury properly could have concluded that Donaldson had been denied his rights simply by comparing the treatment he received while he was under Gumanis's and O'Connor's care with that he received while under Hanenson's care; or it could have concluded that Donaldson's rights had been violated on the basis of the evidence that the defendants obstructed his release even though they knew he was receiving no treatment. Neither judgment required any *a priori* determination of what constitutes or would have constituted adequate treatment, and of course no such determination was made.

We do not, however, concede that determining what constitutes adequate treatment is beyond the competence of the judiciary. In deciding in individual cases whether treatment is adequate, there are a number of devices open to the courts, as Judge Bazelon noted in discussing the implementation of the statutory right to treatment in the landmark case of Rouse v. Cameron:

> But lack of finality [of professional judgment] cannot relieve the court of its duty to render an informed decision. Counsel for the patient and the government can be helpful in presenting pertinent data concerning standards for mental care, and, particularly when the patient is indigent and cannot present experts of his own, the court may appoint independent experts. Assistance might be obtained from such sources as the American Psychiatric Association, which has published standards and is continually engaged in studying the problems of mental care. The court could also consider inviting the psychiatric and legal communities to establish procedures by which expert assistance can be best provided. [Footnotes omitted].

373 F.2d at 457. There are by now many cases where courts have undertaken to determine whether treatment in an individual case is adequate or have ordered that determination to be made by a trial court.[47] Even in cases like *Wyatt* and *Burnham*, when courts are asked to undertake the more difficult task of fashioning institution-wide standards of adequacy, the task should not be beyond them. The experience of the *Wyatt* case bears this out. In *Wyatt*, agreement was reached among the parties on almost all of the minimum standards for adequate treatment ordered by the district court, and the defendants joined in submitting the standards to the district court. These stipulated standards were supported and supplemented by testimony from numerous expert witnesses. Moreover, there was a striking degree of consensus among the experts, including the experts presented by the defendants, as to the minimum standards for adequate treatment. The standards developed have not been challenged by the defendants in the appeal now pending before this Court. See

---

47. See, *e. g.*, Humphrey v. Cady, 1972, 405 U.S. 504, 92 S.Ct. 1048, 31 L.Ed.2d 394; In re Curry, 1971, 147 U.S.App.D.C. 28, 452 F.2d 1360; United States v. Waters, 1970, 141 U.S.App.D.C. 289, 437 F.2d 722; Dobson v. Cameron, 1967, 127 U.S.App.D.C. 324, 383 F.2d 519; Tribby v. Cameron, 126 U.S. App.D.C. 327, 379 F.2d 104; Millard v. Cameron, 1966, 125 U.S.App.D.C. 383, 373 F.2d 468; Sas v. Maryland, 4 Cir. 1964, 334 F.2d 506, remanding, D.Md., 1969, 295 F. Supp. 389, aff'd sub nom., Tippett v. Maryland, 1971, 436 F.2d 1153, cert. dismissed as improvidently granted sub nom., Murel v. Baltimore City Crim.Ct.1972, 407 U.S. 355, 92 S.Ct. 2091, 32 L.Ed.2d 791; Dixon v. Atty. Gen'l of Pennsylvania, M.D.Pa.1971, 325 F.Supp. 966 (three-judge); In re Jones, D.D.C.1972, 338 F.Supp. 428; Clatterbuck v. Harris, D.D.C.1968, 295 F.Supp. 84; Nason v. Supt. of Bridgewater State Hospital, 1968, 353 Mass. 604, 233 N.E.2d 908.

Wyatt v. Stickney, M.D.Ala.1972, 344 F. Supp. 373, 375–376.

In summary, we hold that where a nondangerous patient is involuntarily civilly committed to a state mental hospital, the only constitutionally permissible purpose of confinement is to provide treatment, and that such a patient has a constitutional right to such treatment as will help him to be cured or to improve his mental condition. We hold that the district court did not err in so instructing the jury.

III.

[5] Gumanis and O'Connor join in contending that the evidence at trial did not permit the jury to find that they acted in bad faith, and that therefore they cannot be held personally liable for Donaldson's injuries or the deprivations of his constitutional rights. Gumanis's arguments concern primarily his role in deciding whether Donaldson could or should be released. He asserts that he acted throughout in good faith and in the reasonable belief that Donaldson was mentally ill and required further confinement. O'Connor's argument is directed not only toward his acts affecting the decision whether to release, but also to the entirety of his conduct while Donaldson was held at Florida State. O'Connor argues that both he and Gumanis did the best they could with available resources, and therefore should not be held personally liable for whatever was done to Donaldson. He cites in his brief the various limitations of staff and funds available to the state psychiatrists at Florida State, the difficulties hospital administrators have had in winning approval of their budgets from the state legislatures, and similar matters; and he argues, on that basis, that the denial of whatever right to treatment Donaldson had was the product of the actions of the legislature and of the realities of the budgetary situation, and not of the actions of the state psychia-

trists to whose care Donaldson was entrusted.

We find the appellants' objection, in all of its various forms, without merit. The trial judge instructed the jury:

The defendants in this action rely on the defense that they acted in good faith. Simply put, defendants contend they in good faith believed it was necessary to detain plaintiff in the Florida State Hospital for treatment for the length of time he was so confined. If the jury should believe from a preponderance of the evidence that defendants reasonably believed in good faith the detention of plaintiff was proper for the length of time he was confined then a verdict for defendants should be entered even though the jury may find the detention to have been unlawful.

However, mere good intentions which do not give rise to a reasonable belief that detention is lawfully required cannot justify plaintiff's confinement in the Florida State Hospital. As a corollary plaintiff here need not show malice or ill-will to prove his action under the Civil Rights Act. All that is required is that he demonstrate state action which amounts to an actual deprivation of constitutional rights or other rights guaranteed by law.

The defendants did not object to this instruction, and do not challenge its correctness here.[48] The instruction was proper, and there was sufficient evidence to support a jury finding that the defendants did not act at all times in a good faith and reasonable belief that Donaldson needed continued confinement and that continued confinement was lawful. In effect, the jury found, on the facts, that Donaldson's right to treatment was denied not or not only by the limitations of funds and staff and resources under which the hospital operated, but also by the actions of Gumanis and O'Connor themselves.

48. Dowsey v. Wilkins, 5 Cir 1972, 467 F.2d 1022, 1025–1026.

We are "duty bound to accept all evidence in favor of the verdict as true and to give such evidence the benefit of all permissible inferences that would help sustain the jury's decision". Little v. Green, 5 Cir. 1970, 428 F.2d 1061, cert. denied, 400 U.S. 964, 91 S.Ct. 366, 27 L. Ed.2d 384; Grey v. First National Bank, 5 Cir. 1968, 393 F.2d 371, 381. We hold therefore that the evidence supported the jury's finding that the defendants did not act in good faith.

IV.

The first contention made by Gumanis alone is that the Northern District of Florida's jury selection plan operated to abridge his right to a jury trial under the seventh amendment and under 28 U. S.C. §§ 1861, 1862, by permitting the "systematic exclusion" of physicians from the jury rolls. Gumanis raised his objection to the composition of the jury on the first day of the trial, but after the jury had been impanelled and sworn. The Northern District selection plan allows certain specified classes of person, including "actively engaged members of the clergy" and "actively practicing attorneys, physicians, and dentists, and registered nurses", to be excused from jury duty if they so desire. The authority for these exceptions is an express provision of the Jury Selection and Service Act. 28 U.S.C. § 1863(b)(5) provides that a jury selection plan shall "specify those groups of persons or occupational classes whose member shall, on individual request therefore be excused from jury service. . . . if the district court finds, and the plan states, that jury service by such class or

group would entail undue hardship or extreme inconvenience. . . ."

[6, 7] There is no merit to the defendant's contention. The trial court correctly held that the objection was not timely raised, since the defendants had not mentioned it until after the jury was impanelled. See Brooks v. United States, 5 Cir. 1969, 416 F.2d 1044, 1047. We also agree with his ruling that the jury selection plan was in compliance with the statute.

V.

Gumanis next objects to the trial court's refusal to instruct the jury that Donaldson's claim was barred by the statute of limitations.[49] This contention is premised upon the fact that Donaldson was taken out of his care April 18, 1967, more than four years before the filing of the First Amended Complaint in this case, and about five years before the complaint was amended to add Gumanis as a defendant.

Since there is no statute of limitations provided under § 1983, federal courts adopt the statute of limitations of the state where the action arose,[50] and apply the "resemblance test" to decide which state statute is an appropriate one to apply.[51] In this case, the parties agree that the limitation period should be taken from one of three state statutes: the two-year statute applicable to both false imprisonment actions and to actions for medical malpractice; or the three-year statute applicable to actions upon liabilities created by statute; or the four-year statute applicable to miscellaneous actions not specifically provided for else-

---

49. The instruction in question read:

You are instructed that the statute of limitations for the wrongs alleged in the complaint are for the period of four (4) years, and that the defendants should not be held accountable for any damages which occurred from wrongs occurring prior to the four (4) year period preceding the complaint.

Donaldson argues that the defendants' objection to the trial judge's refusal to give this instruction is not properly before this Court, again because no objection was made

to the trial judge's failure to give the instruction either at the charge conference or after the charge was read to the jury. See note 8 *supra*. Again, however, defendants' pretrial brief advised the court of the defendants' position, and again we hold that that sufficed to excuse the failure to object. See note 8 *supra*.

50. Campbell v. Haverhill, 1895, 155 U.S. 610, 15 S.Ct. 217, 39 L.Ed. 280.

51. See, *e. g.*, Smith v. Cremins, 9 Cir. 1962, 308 F.2d 187.

where in the Florida statute of limitations chapter.[52] Gumanis argues that it is irrelevant which of these 3 periods we apply, since even if the longest, the four-year statute, is applied, the period of limitations had elapsed by the time Gumanis was added as a defendant in this suit. Donaldson agrees that it is irrelevant which statute is chosen, since he argues the limitation did not begin to run until July 31, 1971, the date Donaldson was released from the hospital. Donaldson therefore argues that the suit was timely brought, even if the two-year limitation period applies.

[8–10] We agree with Donaldson that the limitation period, be it two, three, or four years, did not begin to run until July 31; Donaldson's cause of action did not accrue until that time. When a tort involves continuing injury, the cause of action accrues, and the limitation period begins to run, at the time the tortious conduct ceases. See, *e. g.*, Fowkes v. Pennsylvania R. R. Co., 3 Cir. 1959, 264 F.2d 397. In the case of false imprisonment, the tort action this case most resembles, the cause of action does not accrue until the release of the imprisoned party.[53]

[11] We have found no Florida decision addressing the question when a cause of action for false imprisonment accrues. But in a § 1983 suit, even though a state statute is applied, the question when a federal cause of action *accrues* is a matter of federal, not state law.[54] The state statute is applied in the first place not as a matter of legal com-

pulsion, but merely as a matter of convenience; there is no other period of limitation available.[55] We hold that in a case such as this one, where a tort causing continuing injury is alleged, a patient's cause of action does not accrue until the date of his release.

VI.

[12] Gumanis next contends[56] that the district court erred in refusing to instruct the jury that he and the other defendants were entitled to a defense of quasi-judicial immunity under the Civil Rights Acts. At issue is defendant's proposed instruction number 11, which read: "If you find that the defendants were operating in a quasi-judicial function, in that they, under state law, were making a judgment as to whether or not plaintiff should be released, defendants are immune from liability under the Civil Rights Act."

Gumanis relies primarily upon three Ninth Circuit cases. The first and most important is Hoffman v. Halden, 1969, 268 F.2d 280, in which the Ninth Circuit held that the superintendent of a state mental hospital, who allegedly had wrongfully detained a patient committed under a valid judicial commitment order, was immune from liability. The superintendent was empowered to release the patient when, in his own judgment, he found the patient no longer in need of confinement. The Court held that because he had been exercising a "discretionary" function, the Superintendent was immune from liability. The other

---

52. Fla.Stat. § 95.11(4), (5)(a), (6), F.S.A.

53. See, *e. g.*, Bronaugh v. Harding Hospital, Inc., 1958, 12 Ohio App.2d 110, 231 N.E.2d 487; Mobley v. Broome, 1958, 248 N.C. 54, 102 S.E.2d 407; Matovina v. Hult, 1955, 125 Ind.App. 236, 244, 123 N.E.2d 893; Belflower v. Blackshere, Okl.1955, 281 P.2d 423, 425; Oosterwyk v. Bucholtz, 1947, 250 Wis. 521, 525, 27 N.W.2d 361; Jedzierowski v. Jordan, 1961, 157 Me. 352, 172 A.2d 636.

54. See, *e. g.*, Rawlings v. Ray, 1941, 312 U.S. 96, 61 S.Ct. 473, 85 L.Ed. 605; Cope v. Anderson, 1947, 331 U.S. 461, 67 S.Ct. 1340, 91 L.Ed. 1602; Sandidge v. Rogers, S.D.Ind.

1958, 167 F.Supp. 553, 556; 2 Moore's Federal Practice ¶ 3.07(2) at 750.

55. See McAllister v. Magnolia Petroleum Co., 1958, 357 U.S. 221, 228–230, 78 S.Ct. 1201, 2 L.Ed.2d 1272 (Brennan, J., concurring); 2 Moore's Federal Practice ¶ 3.07(2).

56. Once again, Donaldson argues that the objection to the refusal to give the instruction is not properly before the Court. See notes 8, 49 *supra*. Once again, we hold that the trial judge was sufficiently apprised of the defendants' objections for us to consider the objection as having been preserved. See notes 8, 49 *supra*.

two Ninth Circuit cases, Silver v. Dickson, 1968, 403 F.2d 642, and Keeton v. Procunier, 1971, 468 F.2d 810, held that members of state parole boards are immune from § 1983 liability, on the ground that the threat of liability would "exert a restricting influence on the overall functioning of the agency". *Silver*, 403 F.2d at 643.

[13] Gumanis's argument is essentially that he is entitled to the defense, available to state officials in most common law jurisdictions, of absolute immunity for acts done in the performance of a "discretionary"—as opposed to a "ministerial"—function. See, *e. g.*, Barr v. Matteo, 1959, 360 U.S. 564, 79 S.Ct. 1335, 3 L.Ed.2d 1434 (immunity for federal officials as a matter of federal common law). For discussions of the common law rule, see Norton v. McShane, 5 Cir. 1964, 332 F.2d 855, 857–861 (Rives, J.); Anderson v. Nosser, 5 Cir. 1971, 438 F.2d 183, 198–200 (Goldberg, J.), modified en banc on other grounds, 1972, 456 F.2d 835; Carter v. Carlson, 1971, 144 U.S.App.D.C. 388, 447 F.2d 358, 361–365; 2 F. Harper & F. James, The Law of Torts § 29.10 at 1638–46 (1956). We must reject Gumanis's argument, however, because we have consistently held that the full range of officials immunity available at common law do not apply in actions brought under § 1983. Roberts v. Williams, 5 Cir. 1972, 456 F.2d 819, 830; *Anderson, supra*, 438 F.2d at 201; *Norton, supra*, 332 F.2d at 860–861 (dictum). In taking this position we have been joined by all the other circuits that have considered the question. *Carter, supra*, 447 F.2d at 365; Dale v. Hahn, 2 Cir. 1971, 440 F.2d 633; Kletschka v. Driver, 2 Cir. 1969, 411 F.2d 436, 448; Jobson v. Henne, 2 Cir. 1966, 355 F.2d

129, 133–134; McLaughlin v. Tilendis, 7 Cir. 1968, 398 F.2d 287; Donovan v. Reinbold, 9 Cir. 1970, 433 F.2d 738.

Official immunity has been restricted under § 1983, because that provision is directed at actions "under color of any statute, ordinance, regulation, custom, or usage of any State or Territory", and provides that "every person" subjecting another to a deprivation of constitutional rights shall be liable. See Francis v. Lyman, 1 Cir. 1954, 216 F.2d 583, 587; *Jobson, supra*, 355 F.2d at 133; *Anderson, supra*, 438 F.2d at 201; *Hoffman, supra*, 268 F.2d at 300. It has been the view of the courts that recognizing broad judicial immunities "would practically constitute a judicial repeal" of § 1983, since state officers are likely to be the primary persons found acting "under color of" law. *Hoffman, supra*, at 300; *Jobson, supra*, 355 F.2d at 134. Accordingly, the courts have repudiated what the district court for the District of Nevada has called the "discretionary act test" for determining when official immunity is appropriate in § 1983 cases. Adamian v. University of Nevada, 1973, 359 F.Supp. 825, 834. Instead, we and other courts have applied what the *Adamian* court called the "good faith for qualified governmental immunity" test, allowing immunity when (1) the officer's acts were discretionary; *and* (2) the officer was acting in good faith. Here, as noted above, the trial judge instructed the jury to find for the defendants if it found the defendants acted in good faith; and, again as noted above, the defendants have not challenged the propriety or phrasing of this instruction.[57] That instruction was all that was required by this Court's version of the doctrine of "quasi-judicial" or "official" immunity from Civil Rights Act liability.[58]

---

57. The full instruction is quoted in part III *supra*.

58. It is appropriate to say in this context that we do not view the *Hoffman, Silver* and *Keeton* cases as sound authority for a contrary result. The Ninth Circuit has

made it clear that *Hoffman* and *Silver* do not "stand for the broad principle that all public officials are immune from Civil Rights Act liability if their acts were discretionary and done within the scope of their official duties". Donovan v. Reinbold, 9 Cir. 1970, 433 F.2d 738, 744. The Second Cir-

VII.

[14] The remainder of the objections Gumanis raises pose little difficulty. Gumanis contends that the trial judge erred in allowing the jury to award punitive damages. The objection is without merit. The trial judge instructed the jury that it could award punitive damages if it found that the defendants had acted "maliciously", "wantonly", or "oppressively". The instruction was proper as a matter of law, and there was ample evidence, some of it recited in our statement of facts above, to support a jury finding that the defendants' acts were "malicious", "wanton", or "oppressive".

[15] Gumanis argues that Donaldson's failure to receive treatment was a result largely of his own refusal, on religious grounds, to accept certain forms of treatment, particularly medication and electroshock treatments, and his failure to petition for restoration of his competency under Fla. Statutes § 394.22, F.S.A. Neither argument has any merit. As for Donaldson's refusal of forms of treatment, the trial judge instructed the jury: "You are instructed that if Plaintiff through his own actions contributed to the withholding of a particular form of treatment, that Plaintiff is not entitled to collect compensation from the Defendants for the failure to give such treatment during the particular period or periods Plaintiff refused such treatment." Gumanis did not at the trial and does not now object to this instruction. We find no reason to believe that either the verdict or the award of damages was based upon the failure to give Donaldson those forms of treatment he refused. As for his failure to petition for a restoration of his competency, the statute in question does not permit a person adjudged incompetent to petition on his own for a restoration of his competency; the petition may be instituted only by a parent, guardian, or "next friend". Donaldson cannot be held accountable for not doing what he was legally unable to do.

Finally, Gumanis contends that "the cumulative effect of certain errors and irregularities during the course of the trial was such as to significantly undermine the fairness of the trial itself". We have considered these alleged errors too, and find no merit to any one of them. We have also concluded, upon a review of the record, that cumulatively they did not affect the fairness of the trial to any appreciable extent.

The judgment of the district court is

Affirmed.

---

cuit had earlier stated its view that it would have disapproved the *Hoffman* decision if that decision had to be read to mean that "all subordinate state officials should be granted an immunity for all discretionary acts". *Jobson, supra,* 355 F.2d at 134 n. 11. And we ourselves have already once stated our view that *Hoffman* represented a "questionabl[e] resol[ution]" of the problem of official immunity under the Civil Rights Act. Norton v. McShane, 5 Cir. 1964, 332 F.2d 855, 861 n. 9, (Rives, J.). To the extent that *Hoffman*, by implying that state mental health officials should enjoy some form of "quasi-judicial immunity", is read as authority for a result contrary to the one we reach here, we decline to follow it. We rely instead on *Dale* and *Jobson*, where the Second Circuit held state psychiatrists and mental hospital officials were not entitled to immunity under § 1983.

O'Connor v. Donaldson

No. 74–8

| J. B. O'Connor,
Petitioner,
v.
Kenneth Donaldson. | On Writ of Certiorari to the United States Court of Appeals for the Fifth Circuit. |

[June 26, 1975]

MR. JUSTICE STEWART delivered the opinion of the Court.

The respondent, Kenneth Donaldson, was civilly committed to confinement as a mental patient in the Florida State Hospital at Chattahoochee in January of 1957. He was kept in custody there against his will for nearly 15 years. The petitioner, Dr. J. B. O'Connor, was the hospital's superintendent during most of this period. Throughout his confinement Donaldson repeatedly, but unsuccessfully, demanded his release, claiming that he was dangerous to no one, that he was not mentally ill, and that, at any rate, the hospital was not providing treatment for his supposed illness. Finally, in February of 1971, Donaldson brought this lawsuit under 42 U. S. C. § 1983, in the United States District Court for the Northern District of Florida, alleging that O'Connor, and other members of the hospital staff, named as defendants, had intentionally and maliciously deprived him of his constitutional right to liberty.[1] After a four-day trial, the

---

[1] Donaldson's original complaint was filed as a class action on behalf of himself and all of his fellow patients in an entire department of the Florida State Hospital at Chattahoochee. In addition to a damage claim, Donaldson's complaint also asked for habeas corpus relief ordering his release, as well as the release of all members of the

jury returned a verdict assessing both compensatory and punitive damages against O'Connor and a codefendant. The Court of Appeals for the Fifth Circuit affirmed the judgment, 493 F. 2d 507. We granted O'Connor's petition for certiorari, 419 U. S. 894, because of the important constitutional questions seemingly presented.

I

Donaldson's commitment was initiated by his father, who thought that his son was suffering from "delusions." After hearings before a county judge of Pinellas County, Florida, Donaldson was found to be suffering from "paranoid schizophrenia" and was committed for "care, maintenance, and treatment" pursuant to Florida statutory provisions that have since been repealed.[2] The state law

---

class. Donaldson further sought declaratory and injunctive relief requiring the hospital to provide adequate psychiatric treatment.

After Donaldson's release and after the District Court dismissed the action as a class suit, Donaldson filed an amended complaint, repeating his claim for compensatory and punitive damages. Although the amended complaint retained the prayer for declaratory and injunctive relief, that request was eliminated from the case prior to trial. See *Donaldson* v. *O'Connor*, 493 F. 2d 507, 512–513.

[2] The judicial commitment proceedings were pursuant to § 394.22 (11) of the State Public Health Code, which provided:

"Whenever any person who has been adjudged mentally incompetent requires confinement or restraint to prevent self-injury or violence to others, the said judge shall direct that such person be forthwith delivered to a superintendent of a Florida state hospital, for the mentally ill, after admission has been authorized under regulations approved by the board of commissioners of state institutions, for care, maintenance, and treatment, as provided in sections 394.09, 394.24, 394.25, 394.26 and 394.27, or make such other disposition of him as he may be permitted by law . . . ."

1955–1956 Fla. Laws Extra. Sess., c. 31403, § 1, 62.

Donaldson had been adjudged "incompetent" several days earlier under § 394.22 (1), which provided for such a finding as to any person who was

"incompetent by reason of mental illness, sickness, drunkenness,

was less than clear in specifying the grounds necessary for commitment, and the record is scanty as to Donaldson's condition at the time of the judicial hearing. These matters are, however, irrelevant, for this case involves no challenge to the initial commitment, but is focused, instead, upon the nearly 15 years of confinement that followed.

The evidence at the trial showed that the hospital staff had the power to release a patient, not dangerous to himself or others, even if he remained mentally ill

---

excessive use of drugs, insanity, or other mental or physical condition, so that he is incapable of caring for himself or managing his property, or is likely to dissipate or lose his property or become the victim of designing persons, or inflict harm on himself or others . . . ." 1955 Fla. Gen. Laws, c. 29909, § 3, 831.

It would appear that § 394.22 (11)(a) contemplated that involuntary commitment would be imposed only on those "incompetent" persons who "require[d] confinement or restraint to prevent self-injury or violence to others." But this is not certain, for § 394.22 (11)(c) provided that the judge could adjudicate the person a "harmless incompetent" and release him to a guardian upon a finding that he did "not require confinement or restraint to prevent self-injury or violence to others *and* that treatment in the Florida state hospital is unnecessary or would be without benefit to such person . . . ." 1955 Fla. Gen. Laws, c. 29909, § 3, 835 (emphasis added). In this regard, it is noteworthy that Donaldson's "Order for Delivery" to the Florida State Hospital provided that he required "confinement or restraint to prevent self-injury or violence to others, *or* to insure proper treatment." (Emphasis added.) At any rate, the Florida, commitment statute provided no judicial procedure whereby one still incompetent could secure his release on the ground that he was no longer dangerous to himself or others.

Whether the Florida statute provided a "right to treatment" for involuntarily committed patients is also open to dispute. Under § 394.22 (11)(a), commitment "to prevent self-injury or violence to others" was "for care, maintenance, and treatment." Recently Florida has totally revamped its civil commitment law and now provides a statutory right to receive individual medical treatment. 14A Fla. Stat. Ann. § 394.459.

and had been lawfully committed.[3] Despite many requests, O'Connor refused to allow that power to be exercised in Donaldson's case. At the trial, O'Connor indicated that he had believed that Donaldson would have been unable to make a "successful adjustment outside the institution," but could not recall the basis for that conclusion. O'Connor retired as superintendent shortly before this suit was filed. A few months thereafter, and before the trial, Donaldson secured his release and a judicial restoration of competency, with the support of the hospital staff.

The testimony at the trial demonstrated, without contradiction, that Donaldson had posed no danger to others during his long confinement, or indeed at any point in his life. O'Connor himself conceded that he had no personal or secondhand knowledge that Donaldson had ever committed a dangerous act. There was no evidence that Donaldson had ever been suicidal or been thought likely to inflict injury upon himself. One of O'Connor's codefendants acknowledged that Donaldson could have earned

---

[3] The sole *statutory* procedure for release required a judicial reinstatement of a patient's "mental competency." Public Health Code §§ 394.22 (15), (16), 1955 Fla. Gen. Laws c. 29909, § 3, 838–841. But this procedure could be initiated by the hospital staff. Indeed, it was at the staff's initiative that Donaldson was finally restored to competency, and liberty, almost immediately after O'Connor retired from the superintendency.

In addition, witnesses testified that the hospital had always had its own procedure for releasing patients—for "trial visits," "home visits," "furloughs," or "out of state discharges"—even though the patients had not been judicially restored to competency. Those conditional releases often became permanent, and the hospital merely closed its books on the patient. O'Connor did not deny at trial that he had the power to release patients; he conceded that it was his "duty" as superintendent of the hospital "to determine whether that patient having once reached the hospital was in such condition as to request that he be considered for release from the hospital."

his own living outside the hospital. He had done so for some 14 years before his commitment, and immediately upon his release he secured a responsible job in hotel administration.

Furthermore, Donaldson's frequent requests for release had been supported by responsible persons willing to provide him any care he might need on release. In 1963, for example, a representative of Helping Hands, Inc., a halfway house for mental patients, wrote O'Connor asking him to release Donaldson to its care. The request was accompanied by a supporting letter from the Minneapolis Clinic of Psychiatry and Neurology, which a codefendant conceded was a "good clinic." O'Connor rejected the offer, replying that Donaldson could be released only to his parents. That rule was apparently of O'Connor's own making. At the time, Donaldson was 55 years old, and, as O'Connor knew, Donaldson's parents were too elderly and infirm to take responsibiltiy for him. Moreover, in his continuing correspondence with Donaldson's parents, O'Connor never informed them of the Helping Hands offer. In addition, on four separate occasions between 1964 and 1968, John Lembcke, a college classmate of Donaldson's and a longtime family friend, asked O'Connor to release Donaldson to his care. On each occasion O'Connor refused. The record shows that Lembcke was a serious and responsible person, who was willing and able to assume responsibility for Donaldson's welfare.

The evidence showed that Donaldson's confinement was a simple regime of enforced custodial care, not a program designed to alleviate or cure his supposed illness. Numerous witnesses, including one of O'Connor's codefendants, testified that Donaldson had received nothing but custodial care while at the hospital. O'Connor described Donaldson's treatment as "milieu therapy."

But witnesses from the hospital staff conceded that, in the context of this case, "milieu therapy" was a euphemism for confinement in the "milieu" of a mental hospital.[4] For substantial periods, Donaldson was simply kept in a large room that housed 60 patients, many of whom were under criminal commitment. Donaldson's requests for ground privileges, occupational training, and an opportunity to discuss his case with O'Connor or other staff members were repeatedly denied.

At the trial, O'Connor's principal defense was that he had acted in good faith and was therefore immune from any liability for monetary damages. His position, in short, was that state law, which he had believed valid, had authorized indefinite custodial confinement of the "sick," even if they were not given treatment and their release could harm no one.[5]

The trial judge instructed the members of the jury that they should find that O'Connor had violated Donaldson's constitutional right to liberty if they found that he had

"confined [Donaldson] against his will, knowing that he was not mentally ill or dangerous or knowing that

---

[4] There was some evidence that Donaldson, who is a Christian Scientist, on occasion refused to take medication. The trial judge instructed the jury not to award damages for any period of confinement during which Donaldson had declined treatment.

[5] At the close of Donaldson's case-in-chief, O'Connor moved for a directed verdict on the ground that state law at the time of Donaldson's confinement authorized institutionalization of the mentally ill even if they posed no danger to themselves or others. This motion was denied. At the close of all the evidence, O'Connor asked that the jury be instructed that "if the defendants acted pursuant to a statute which was not declared unconstitutional at the time, they cannot be held accountable for such action." The District Court declined to give this requested instruction.

if mentally ill he was not receiving treatment for his mental illness . . . .

. . . . .

"Now the purpose of involuntary hospitalization is treatment and not mere custodial care or punishment if a patient is not a danger to himself or others. Without such treatment there is no justification from a constitutional standpoint for continued confinement unless you should also find that [Donaldson] was dangerous either to himself or others." [6]

---

[6] The District Court defined treatment as follows:

"You are instructed that a person who is involuntarily civilly committed to a mental hospital does have a constitutional right to receive such treatment *as will give him a realistic opportunity to be cured or to improve his mental condition.*" (Emphasis added.)

O'Connor argues that this statement suggests that a mental patient has a right to treatment even if confined by reason of dangerousness to himself or others. But this is to take the above paragraph out of context, for it is bracketed by paragraphs making clear the trial judge's theory that treatment is constitutionally required only if mental illness alone, rather than danger to self or others, is the reason for confinement. If O'Connor had thought the instructions ambiguous on this point, he could have objected to them and requested a clarification. He did not do so. We accordingly have no occasion here to decide whether persons committed on grounds of dangerousness enjoy a "right to treatment."

In pertinent part, the instructions read as follows:

"The Plaintiff claims in brief that throughout the period of his hospitalization he was not mentally ill or dangerous to himself or others, and claims further that if he was mentally ill, or if Defendants believed he was mentally ill, Defendants withheld from him the treatment necessary to improve his mental condition.

"The Defendants claim, in brief, that Plaintiff's detention was legal and proper, or if his detention was not legal and proper, it was the result of mistake, without malicious intent.

. . . . .

"In order to prove his claim under the Civil Rights Act, the burden is upon the Plaintiff in this case to establish by a preponderance of the evidence in this case the following facts:

"That the Defendants confined Plaintiff against his will, know-

The trial judge further instructed the jury that O'Connor was immune from damages if he

> "reasonably believed in good faith that detention of [Donaldson] was proper for the length of time he was so confined . . . .
>
> "However, mere good intentions which do not give rise to a reasonable belief that detention is lawfully required cannot justify [Donaldson's] confinement in the Florida State Hospital."

The jury returned a verdict for Donaldson against O'Connor and a codefendant, and awarded damages of $38,500, including $10,000 in punitive damages.[7]

The Court of Appeals affirmed the judgment of the District Court in a broad opinion dealing with "the far-reaching question whether the Fourteenth Amendment guarantees a right to treatment to persons involuntarily

---

ing that he was not mentally ill or dangerous or knowing that if mentally ill he was not receiving treatment for his mental illness.

.   .   .   .   .

"[T]hat the Defendants' acts and conduct deprived the Plaintiff of his Federal Constitutional right not to be denied or deprived of his liberty without due process of law as that phrase is defined and explained in these instructions . . . .

.   .   .   .   .

"You are instructed that a person who is involuntarily civilly committed to a mental hospital does have a constitutional right to receive such treatment as will give him a realistic opportunity to be cured or to improve his mental condition.

"Now the purpose of involuntary hospitalization is treatment and not mere custodial care or punishment if a patient is not a danger to himself or others. Without such, treatment there is no justification from a constitutional stand-point for continued confinement unless you should also find that the Plaintiff was dangerous either to himself or others."

[7] The trial judge had instructed that punitive damages should be awarded only if "the act or omission of the Defendant or Defendants which proximately caused injury to the Plaintiff was maliciously or wantonly or oppressively done."

civilly committed to state mental hospitals." 493 F. 2d, at 509. The appellate court held that when, as in Donaldson's case, the rationale for confinement is that the patient is in need of treatment, the Constitution requires that minimally adequate treatment in fact be provided. *Id.,* at 521. The court further expressed the view that, regardless of the grounds for involuntary civil commitment, a person confined against his will at a state mental institution has "a constitutional right to receive such individual treatment as will give him a reasonable opportunity to be cured or to improve his mental condition." *Id.,* at 520. Conversely, the court's opinion implied that it is constitutionally permissible for a State to confine a mentally ill person against his will in order to treat his illness, regardless of whether his illness renders him dangerous to himself or others. See *id.,* at 522–527.

II

We have concluded that the difficult issues of constitutional law dealt with by the Court of Appeals are not presented by this case in its present posture. Specifically, there is no reason now to decide whether mentally ill persons dangerous to themselves or to others have a right to treatment upon compulsory confinement by the State, or whether the State may compulsorily confine a nondangerous, mentally ill individual for the purpose of treatment. As we view it, this case raises a single, relatively simple, but nonetheless important question concerning every man's constitutional right to liberty.

The jury found that Donaldson was neither dangerous to himself nor dangerous to others, and also found that, if mentally ill, Donaldson had not received treatment.[8]

---

[8] Given the jury instructions, see n. 6 *supra,* it is possible that the jury went so far as to find that O'Connor knew not only that Donaldson was harmless to himself and others but also that he was

That verdict, based on abundant evidence, makes the issue before the Court a narrow one. We need not decide whether, when, or by what procedures, a mentally ill person may be confined by the State on any of the grounds which, under contemporary statutes, are generally advanced to justify involuntary confinement of such a person—to prevent injury to the public, to ensure his own survival or safety,[9] or to alleviate or cure his illness. See *Jackson* v. *Indiana,* 406 U. S. 715, 736–737; *Humphrey* v. *Cady,* 405 U. S. 504, 509. For the jury found that none of the above grounds for continued confinement was present in Donaldson's case.[10]

---

not mentally ill at all. If it so found, the jury was permitted by the instructions to rule against O'Connor regardless of the nature of the "treatment" provided. If we were to construe the jury's verdict in that fashion, there would remain no substantial issue in this case: That a wholly sane and innocent person has a constitutional right not to be physically confined by the State when his freedom will pose a danger neither to himself nor to others cannot be seriously doubted.

[9] The judge's instructions used the phrase "dangerous to himself." Of course, even if there is no foreseeable risk of self-injury or suicide, a person is literally "dangerous to himself" if for physical or other reasons he is helpless to avoid the hazards of freedom either through his own efforts or with the aid of willing family members or friends. While it might be argued that the judge's instructions could have been more detailed on this point, O'Connor raised no objection to them, presumably because the evidence clearly showed that Donaldson was not "dangerous to himself" however broadly that phrase might be defined.

[10] O'Connor argues that, despite the jury's verdict, the Court must assume that Donaldson was receiving treatment sufficient to justify his confinement, because the adequacy of treatment is a "nonjusticiable" question that must be left to the discretion of the psychiatric profession. That argument is unpersuasive. Where "treatment" is the sole asserted ground for depriving a person of liberty, it is plainly unacceptable to suggest that the courts are powerless to determine whether the asserted ground is present. See *Jackson* v. *Indiana, supra.* Neither party objected to the jury in-

Given the jury's findings, what was left as justification for keeping Donaldson in continued confinement? The fact that state law may have authorized confinement of the harmless mentally ill does not itself establish a constitutionally adequate purpose for the confinement. See *Jackson* v. *Indiana, supra,* at 720–723; *McNeil* v. *Director, Patuxent Institution,* 407 U. S. 245, 248–250. Nor is it enough that Donaldson's original confinement was founded upon a constitutionally adequate basis, if in fact it was, because even if his involuntary confinement was initially permissible, it could not constitutionally continue after that basis no longer existed. *Jackson* v. *Indiana, supra,* at 738; *McNeil* v. *Director, Patuxent Institution, supra.*

A finding of "mental illness" alone cannot justify a State's locking a person up against his will and keeping him indefinitely in simple custodial confinement. Assuming that that term can be given a reasonably precise content and that the "mentally ill" can be identified with reasonable accuracy, there is still no constitutional basis for confining such persons involuntarily if they are dangerous to no one and can live safely in freedom.

May the State confine the mentally ill merely to ensure them a living standard superior to that they enjoy in the private community? That the State has a proper interest in providing care and assistance to the unfortunate goes without saying. But the mere presence of mental illness does not disqualify a person from preferring his home to the comforts of an institution.

---

struction defining treatment. There is, accordingly, no occasion in this case to decide whether the provision of treatment, standing alone, can ever constitutionally justify involuntary confinement or, if it can, how much or what kind of treatment would suffice for that purpose. In its present posture this case involves not involuntary treatment but simply involuntary custodial confinement.

Moreover, while the State may arguably confine a person to save him from harm, incarceration is rarely if ever a necessary condition for raising the living standards of those capable of surviving safely in freedom, on their own or with the help of family or friends. See *Shelton* v. *Tucker,* 364 U. S. 479, 488–490.

May the State fence in the harmless mentally ill solely to save its citizens from exposure to those whose ways are different? One might as well ask if the State, to avoid public unease, could incarcerate all who are physically unattractive or socially eccentric. Mere public intolerance or animosity cannot constitutionally justify the deprivation of a person's physical liberty. See, *e. g., Cohen* v. *California,* 403 U. S. 15, 24–26; *Coates* v. *City of Cincinnati,* 402 U. S. 611, 615; *Street* v. *New York,* 394 U. S. 576, 592; cf. *United States Dept. of Agric.* v. *Moreno,* 413 U. S. 528, 534.

In short, a State cannot constitutionally confine without more a nondangerous individual who is capable of surviving safely in freedom by himself or with the help of willing and responsible family members or friends. Since the jury found, upon ample evidence, that O'Connor, as an agent of the State, knowingly did so confine Donaldson, it properly concluded that O'Connor violated Donaldson's constitutional right to freedom.

III

O'Connor contends that in any event he should not be held personally liable for monetary damages because his decisions were made in "good faith." Specifically, O'Connor argues that he was acting pursuant to state law which, he believed, authorized confinement of the mentally ill even when their release would not compromise their safety or constitute a danger to others, and that he could not reasonably have been expected to know that the state law as he understood it was constitutionally invalid. A proposed instruction to this effect was rejected by the District Court.[11]

The District Court did instruct the jury, without objection, that monetary damages could not be assessed against O'Connor if he had believed reasonably and in good faith that Donaldson's continued confinement was "proper," and that punitive damages could be awarded only if O'Connor had acted "maliciously or wantonly or oppressively." The Court of Appeals approved those instructions. But that court did not consider whether it was error for the trial judge to refuse the additional instruction concerning O'Connor's claimed reliance on state law as authorization for Donaldson's continued confinement. Further, neither the District Court nor the Court of Appeals acted with the benefit of this Court's most recent decision on the scope of the qualified immunity possessed by state officials under 42 U. S. C. § 1983. *Wood* v. *Strickland,* —— U. S. ——.

Under that decision, the relevant question for the jury is whether O'Connor "knew or reasonably should have known that the action he took within his sphere of official responsibility would violate the constitutional rights of [Donaldson], or if he took the action with the malicious intention to cause a deprivation of constitutional rights or other injury to [Donaldson]." *Id.,* ——. See also *Scheuer* v. *Rhodes,* 416 U. S. 232, 247–248; *Wood* v. *Strickland, supra,* at —— (opinion of POWELL, J.). For

---

[11] See n. 5, *supra.* During his years of confinement, Donaldson unsuccessfully petitioned the state and federal courts for release from the Florida State Hospital on a number of occasions. None of these claims was ever resolved on its merits, and no evidentiary hearings were ever held. O'Connor has not contended that he relied on these unsuccessful court actions as an independent intervening reason for continuing Donaldson's confinement, and no instructions on this score were requested.

purposes of this question, an official has, of course, no duty to anticipate unforeseeable constitutional developments. *Wood* v. *Strickland, supra,* at ——.

Accordingly, we vacate the judgment of the Court of Appeals and remand the case to enable that court to consider, in light of *Wood* v. *Strickland,* whether the District Judge's failure to instruct with regard to the effect of O'Connor's claimed reliance on state law rendered inadequate the instructions as to O'Connor's liability for compensatory and punitive damages.[12]

It is so ordered.

---

[12] Upon remand, the Court of Appeals is to consider only the question whether O'Connor is to be held liable for monetary damages for violating Donaldson's constitutional right to liberty. The jury found, on substantial evidence and under adequate instructions, that O'Connor deprived Donaldson, who was dangerous neither to himself nor to others and was provided no treatment, of the constitutional right to liberty. Cf. n. 8, *supra.* That fiinding needs no further consideration. If the Court of Appeals holds that a remand to the District Court is necessary, the only issue to be determined in that court will be whether O'Connor is immune from liability for monetary damages.

Of necessity our decision vacating the judgment of the Court of Appeals deprives that court's opinion of precedential effect, leaving this Court's opinion and judgment as the sole law of the case. See *United States* v. *Munsingwear,* 340 U. S. 36.

SUPREME COURT OF THE UNITED STATES

No. 74-8

J. B. O'Connor,
Petitioner,

v.

Kenneth Donaldson.

On Writ of Certiorari to the
United States Court of Appeals
for the Fifth Circuit.

[June 26, 1975]

MR. CHIEF JUSTICE BURGER, concurring.

Although I join the Court's opinion and judgment in this case, it seems to me that several factors merit more emphasis than it gives them. I therefore add the following remarks.

I

With respect to the remand to the Court of Appeals on the issue of official immunity,[1] it seems to me not entirely irrelevant that there was substantial evidence that Donaldson consistently refused treatment that was offered to him, claiming that he was not mentally ill and needed no treatment.[2] The Court appropriately takes notice of the uncertainties of

---

[1] I have difficulty understanding how the issue of immunity can be resolved on this record and hence it is very likely a new trial may be required; if that is the case I would hope these sensitive and important issues would have the benefit of more effective presentation and articulation on behalf of petitioner.

[2] The Court's reference to "milieu therapy," *ante,* at 5, may be construed as disparaging that concept. True, it is capable of being used simply to cloak official indifference, but the reality is that some mental abnormalities respond to no known treatment. Also some mental patients respond, as do persons suffering from a variety of physiological ailments, to what is loosely called "milieu treatment," *i. e.,* keeping them comfortable, well-nourished, and in a protected environment. It is not for us to say in the baffling field of psychiatry that "milieu therapy" is always a pretense.

psychiatric diagnosis and therapy, and the reported cases are replete with evidence of the divergence of medical opinion in this vexing area. *E. g., Greenwood* v. *United States,* 350 U. S. 366, 375 (1957). See also *Drope* v. *Missouri* — U. S. — (1975). Nonetheless, one of the few areas of agreement among behaviorial specialists is that an uncooperative patient cannot benefit from therapy and that the first step in effective treatment is acknowledgement by the patient that he is suffering from an abnormal condition. See, *e. g.,* Katz, The Right to Treatment—An Enchanting Legal Fiction? 36 U. Chi. L. Rev. 755, 768–769 (1969). Donaldson's adamant refusal to do so should be taken into account in considering petitioner's good-faith defense.

Perhaps more important to the issue of immunity is a factor referred to only obliquely in the Court's opinion. On numerous occasions during the period of his confinement Donaldson unsuccessfully sought release in the Florida courts; indeed, the last of these proceedings was terminated only a few months prior to the bringing of this action. See *Donaldson* v. *O'Connor,* 234 So. 2d 114 (Fla.), cert. denied, 400 U. S. 869 (1970). Whatever the reasons for the state courts' repeated denials of relief, and regardless of whether they correctly resolved the issue tendered to them, petitioner and the other members of the medical staff at Florida State Hospital would surely have been justified in considering each such judicial decision as an approval of continued confinement and an independent intervening reason for continuing Donaldson's confinement. Thus, this fact is inescapably related to the issue of immunity and must be considered by the Court of Appeals on remand and, if a new trial is ordered, by the District Court.[3]

---

[3] That petitioner's counsel failed to raise this issue is not a reason why it should not be considered with respect to immunity in light

II

As the Court points out, *ante*, at 7 n. 6, the District Court instructed the jury in part that "a person who is involuntarily civilly committed to a mental hospital does have a *constitutional* right to receive such treatment as will give him a realistic opportunity to be cured," (emphasis added) and the Court of Appeals unequivocally approved this phrase, standing alone, as a correct statement of the law. *O'Connor* v. *Donaldson*, 493 F. 2d 507, 520 (CA5 1974). The Court's opinion plainly gives no approval to that holding and makes clear that it binds neither the parties to this case nor the courts of the Fifth Circuit. See *ante*, at 14 n. 12. Moreover, in light of its importance for future litigation in this area, it should be emphasized that the Court of Appeals' analysis has no basis in the decisions of this Court.

A

There can be no doubt that involuntary commitment to a mental hospital, like involuntary confinement of an individual for any reason, is a deprivation of liberty which the State cannot accomplish without due process of law. *Specht* v. *Patterson*, 386 U. S., at 608. Cf. *In re Gault*, 387 U. S. 1, 12–13 (1967). Commitment must be justified on the basis of a legitimate state interest, and the reasons for committing a particular individual must be established in an appropriate proceeding. Equally important, confinement must cease when those reasons no longer exist. See *McNeil* v. *Director, Patuxent Institution*, 407 U. S., at 249–250; *Jackson* v. *Indiana*, 406 U. S., at 738.

The Court of Appeals purported to be applying these principles in developing the first of its theories support-

of the Court's holding that the defense was preserved for appellate review.

ing a constitutional right to treatment. It first identified what it perceived to be the traditional bases for civil commitment—physical dangerousness to oneself or others, or a need for treatment—and stated:

> "[W]here, as in Donaldson's case, the rationale for confinement is the *'parens patriae'* rationale that the patient is in need of treatment, the due process clause requires that minimally adequate treatment be in fact provided . . . . 'To deprive any citizen of his or her liberty upon the altruistic theory that the confinement is for humane therapeutic reasons and then fail to provide adequate treatment violates the very fundamentals of due process." 493 F. 2d, at 521.

The Court of Appeals did not explain its conclusion that the rationale for respondent's commitment was that he needed treatment. The Florida statutes in effect during the period of his confinement did not require that a person who had been adjudicated incompetent and ordered committed either be provided with psychiatric treatment or released, and there was no such condition in respondent's order of commitment. Cf. *Rouse* v. *Cameron*, —— U. S. App. D. C. ——, 373 F. 2d 451 (1966). More important, the instructions which the Court of Appeals read as establishing an absolute constitutional right to treatment did not require the jury to make any findings regarding the specific reasons for respondent's confinement or to focus upon any rights he may have had under state law. Thus, the premise of the Court of Appeals' first theory must have been that, at least with respect to persons who are not physically dangerous, a State has no power to confine the mentally ill except for the purpose of providing them with treatment.

That proposition is surely not descriptive of the power traditionally exercised by the States in this area.

Historically, and for a considerable period of time, subsidized custodial care in private foster homes or boarding houses was the most benign form of care provided incompetent or mentally ill persons for whom the States assumed responsibility. Until well into the 19th century the vast majority of such persons were simply restrained in poorhouses, almshouses, or jails. See A. Deutsch, The Mentally Ill in America 38–54, 114–131 (2d ed. 1949). The few States that established institutions for the mentally ill during this early period were concerned primarily with providing a more humane place of confinement and only secondarily with "curing" the persons sent there. See *id.*, at 98–113.

As the trend toward state care of the mentally ill expanded, eventually leading to the present statutory schemes for protecting such persons, the dual functions of institutionalization continued to be recognized. While one of the goals of this movement was to provide medical treatment to those who could benefit from it, it was acknowledged that this could not be done in all cases and that there was a large range of mental illness for which no known "cure" existed. In time, providing places for the custodial confinement of the so-called "dependent insane" again emerged as the major goal of the State's programs in this area and continued to be so well into this century. See *id.*, at 228–271; D. Rothman, The Discovery of the Asylum 264–295 (1971).

In short, the idea that States may not confine the mentally ill except for the purpose of providing them with treatment is of very recent origin,[4] and there is no historical basis for imposing such a limitation on state power. Analysis of the sources of the civil commitment power likewise lends no support to that notion. There can be little doubt that in the exercise of its police power

---

[4] See Editorial, A New Right, 46 A. B. A. J. 516 (1960).

a State may confine individuals solely to protect society from the dangers of significant antisocial acts or communicable disease. Cf. *Minnesota ex rel. Pearson* v. *Probate Court,* 309 U. S. 270; *Jacobson* v. *Massachusetts,* 197 U. S. 1, 25–29 (1905). Additionally, the States are vested with the historic *parens patriae* power, including the duty to protect "persons under legal disabilities to act for themselves." *Hawaii* v. *Standard Oil Co.,* 405 U. S. 251, 257 (1972). See also *Mormon Church* v. *United States,* 136 U. S. 1, 56–58 (1890). The classic example of this role is when a State undertakes to act as " 'the general guardian of all infants, idiots, and lunatics." *Hawaii* v. *Standard Oil Co., supra,* quoting 3 W. Blackstone, Commentaries *47.

Of course, an inevitable consequence of exercising the *parens patriae* power is that the ward's personal freedom will be substantially restrained, whether a guardian is appointed to control his property, he is placed in the custody of a private third party, or committed to an institution. Thus, however the power is implemented, due process requires that it not be invoked indiscriminately. At a minimum, a particular scheme for protection of the mentally ill must rest upon a legislative determination that it is compatible with the best interests of the affected class and that its members are unable to act for themselves. Cf. *Mormon Church* v. *United States, supra.* Moreover, the use of alternative forms of protection may be motivated by different considerations, and the justifications for one may not be invoked to rationalize another. Cf. *Jackson* v. *Indiana,* 406 U. S., at 737–738. See also American Bar Foundation, The Mentally Disabled and the Law, 254–255 (S. Brakel & R. Rock ed. 1971).

However, the existence of some due process limitations on the *parens patriae* power does not justify the further conclusion that it may be exercised to confine a mentally ill person only if the purpose of the confinement is treatment. Despite many recent advances in medical knowledge, it remains a stubborn fact that there are many forms of mental illness which are not understood, some which are untreatable in the sense that no effective therapy has yet been discovered for them, and that rates of "cure" are generally low. See Schwitzgebel, The Right to Effective Mental Treatment, 62 Calif. L. Rev. 936, 941–948 (1974). There can be little responsible debate regarding "the uncertainty of diagnosis in this field and the tentativeness of professional judgment." *Greenwood* v. *United States*, 350 U. S. 366, 375 (1957). See also Ennis and Litwack, Psychiatry and the Presumption of Expertise: Flipping Coins in the Courtroom, 62 Calif. L. Rev. 693, 697–719 (1974).[5] Similarly, as previously observed, it is universally recognized as fundamental to effective therapy that the patient acknowledge his illness and cooperate with those attempting to give treatment; yet the failure of a large proportion of mentally ill persons to do so is a common phenomenon. See Katz, *supra*, 36 U. Chi. L. Rev., at 768–769 (1969). It may be that some persons in either of these categories,[6] and there may be others, are unable to function in society and will suffer real harm to themselves unless provided with care in a sheltered environment. See, *e. g.*, *Lake* v. *Cameron*, —— U. S. App. D. C.

---

[5] Indeed, there is considerable debate concerning the threshold questions of what constitutes "mental disease" and "treatment." See Szasz, The Right to Health, 57 Geo. L. J. 734 (1969).

[6] Indeed, respondent may have shared both of these characteristics. His illness, paranoid schizophrenia, is notoriously unsusceptible to treatment, see Livermore, Malmquist, and Meehl, On the Justifications for Civil Commitment, 117 U. Pa. L. Rev. 75, 93 & n. 52 (1968), and the reports of the Florida State Hospital Staff which were introduced into evidence expressed the view that he was unwilling to acknowledge his illness and generally uncooperative.

—, 364 F. 2d 657, 663–664 (1966) (dissenting opinion). At the very least, I am not able to say that a state legislature is powerless to make that kind of judgment. See *Greenwood* v. *United States, supra.*

B

Alternatively, it has been argued that a Fourteenth Amendment right to treatment for involuntarily confined mental patients derives from the fact that many of the safeguards of the criminal process are not present in civil commitment. The Court of Appeals described this theory as follows:

> "[A] due process right to treatment is based on the principle that when the three central limitations on the government's power to detain—that detention be in retribution for a specific offense; that it be limited to a fixed term; and that it be permitted after a proceeding where the fundamental procedural safeguards are observed—are absent, there must be a *quid pro quo* extended by the government to justify confinement. And the *quid pro quo* most commonly recognized is the provision of rehabilitative treatment." 493 F. 2d, at 522.

To the extent that this theory may be read to permit a State to confine an individual simply because it is willing to provide treatment, regardless of the subject's ability to function in society, it raises the gravest of constitutional problems, and I have no doubt the Court of Appeals would agree on this score. As a justification for a constitutional right to such treatment, the *quid pro quo* theory suffers from equally serious defects.

It is too well established to require extended discussion that due process is not an inflexible concept. Rather, its requirements are determined in particular instances by identifying and accommodating the interests of the individual and society. See, *e. g., Morrissey* v. *Brewer,* 408 U. S. 471, 480–484 (1972); *McNeil* v. *Director, Patuxent Institution,* 407 U. S., at 249–250; *McKeiver* v. *Pennsylvania,* 403 U. S. 528, 545–555 (1971). Where claims that the State is acting in the best interests of an individual are said to justify reduced procedural and substantive safeguards, this Court's decisions require that they be "candidly appraised." *In re Gault,* 387 U. S., at 21, 27–29. However, in so doing judges are not free to read their private notions of public policy or public health into the Constitution. *Olsen* v. *Nebraska,* 313 U. S. 236, 246–247 (1941).

The *quid pro quo* theory is a sharp departure from, and cannot coexist with, these due process principles. As an initial matter, the theory presupposes that essentially the same interests are involved in every situation where a State seeks to confine an individual; that assumption, however, is incorrect. It is elementary that the justification for the criminal process and the unique deprivation of liberty which it can impose requires that it be invoked only for commission of a specific offense prohibited by legislative enactment. See *Powell* v. *Texas,* 392 U. S. 514, 541–544 (1968) (opinion of Black, J.).[7] But it would be incongruous to apply the same limitation when quarantine is imposed by the State to protect the public from a highly communicable disease. See *Jacobson* v. *Massachusetts,* 197 U. S., at 29–30.

---

[7] This is not to imply that I accept all of the Court of Appeals' conclusions regarding the limitations upon the States' power to detain persons who commit crimes. For example, the notion that confinement must be "for a fixed term" is difficult to square with the widespread practice of indeterminate sentencing, at least where the upper limit is life.

A more troublesome feature of the *quid pro quo* theory is that it elevates a concern for essentially procedural safeguards into a new substantive constitutional right.[8] Rather than inquiring whether strict standards of proof or periodic redetermination of a patient's condition are required in civil confinement, the theory accepts the absence of such safeguards but insists that the State provide benefits which, in the view of a court, are adequate "compensation" for confinement. In light of the wide divergence of medical opinion regarding the diagnosis of and proper therapy for mental abnormalities, that prospect is especially troubling in this area and cannot be squared with the principle that "courts may not substitute for the judgments of legislators their own understanding of the public welfare, but must instead concern themselves with the validity of the methods which the legislature has selected." *In re Gault*, 387 U. S., at 71 (opinion of Harlan, J.). Of course, questions regarding the adequacy of procedure and the power of a State to continue particular confinements are ultimately for the courts, aided by expert opinion to the extent that is found helpful. But I am not persuaded that we should abandon the traditional limitations on the scope of judicial review.

C

In sum, I cannot accept the reasoning of the Court of Appeals and can discern no other basis for equating an involuntarily committed mental patient's unquestioned constitutional right not to be confined without due process of law with a constitutional right to *treatment*.[9]

[8] Even advocates of a right to treatment have criticized the *quid pro quo* theory on this ground. *E. g.*, Note, Developments in the Law—Civil Commitment of the Mentally Ill, 87 Harv. L. Rev. 1190, 1325, n. 39 (1974).

[9] It should be pointed out that several issues which the Court has touched upon in other contexts are not involved here. As

Given the present state of medical knowledge regarding abnormal human behavior and its treatment, few things would be more fraught with peril than to irrevocably condition a State's power to protect the mentally ill upon the providing of "such treatment as will give [them] a realistic opportunity to be cured." Nor can I accept the theory that a State may lawfully confine an individual thought to need treatment and justify that deprivation

---

the Court's opinion makes plain, this is not a case of a person seeking release because he has been confined "without ever obtaining a judicial determination that such confinement is warranted." *McNeil* v. *Director, Patuxent Institution,* 407 U. S. 245, 249 (1972). Although respondent's amended complaint alleged that his 1956 hearing before the Pinellas County Court was procedurally defective and ignored various factors relating to the necessity for commitment, the persons to whom those allegations applied were either not served with process or dismissed by the District Court prior to trial. Respondent has not sought review of the latter rulings, and this case does not involve the rights of a person in an initial competency or commitment proceeding. Cf. *Jackson* v. *Indiana,* 406 U. S. 715, 738 (1972); *Specht* v. *Patterson,* 386 U. S. 605 (1967); *Minnesota ex rel. Pearson* v. *Probate Court,* 309 U. S. 270 (1940).

Further, it was not alleged that respondent was singled out for discriminatory treatment by the staff of Florida State Hospital or that patients at that institution were denied privileges generally available to other persons under commitment in Florida. Thus, the question whether different bases for commitment justify differences in conditions of confinement is not involved in this litigation. Cf. *Jackson* v. *Indiana, supra,* at 723–730; *Baxstrom* v. *Herold,* 383 U. S. 107 (1966).

Finally, there was no evidence whatever that respondent was abused or mistreated at Florida State Hospital or that the failure to provide him with treatment aggravated his condition. There was testimony regarding the general quality of life at the hospital, but the jury was not asked to consider whether respondent's confinement was in effect "punishment" for being mentally ill. The record provides no basis for concluding, therefore, that respondent was denied rights secured by the Eighth and Fourteenth Amendments. Cf. *Robinson* v. *California,* 370 U. S. 660 (1962).

of liberty solely by providing some treatment. Our concepts of due process would not tolerate such a "trade-off." Because the Court of Appeals' analysis could be read as authorizing those results, it should not be followed.

Appendix A

CONFERENCE PARTICIPANTS

BENJAMIN BRAGINSKY
Professor of Psychology,
Wesleyan University,
Middletown, Conn.

ALEXANDER BROOKS
Professor of Law,
Rutgers Law School,
Newark, N. J.

GALEN BURGHARDT
Assistant Professor of Economics,
University of Massachusetts,
Amherst, Mass.

ARTHUR CENTOR
Administrative Officer for Professional Affairs,
American Psychological Association,
Washington, D. C.

JULIUS COHEN
Institute for the Study of Mental Retardation
 and Related Disabilities,
University of Michigan,
Ann Arbor, Mich.

OLIVER FOWLKES
Assistant Professor of Law,
Hampshire College,
Amherst, Mass.

WILLIAM FREMOUW
Assistant Professor of Psychology,
West Virginia University,
Morgantown, West Va.

WILLIAM GOGGINS
Business Manager,
Northampton State Hospital,
Northampton, Mass.

STUART GOLANN
Professor of Psychology,
University of Massachusetts,
Amherst, Mass.

CHARLES HALPERN
Attorney,
Center for Law and Social Policy,
Washington, D. C.

WILLIAM JONES
Superintendent,
Belchertown State School,
Belchertown, Mass.

MARION LANGER
Executive Director,
American Orthopsychiatric Association,
New York, N. Y.

THE HONORABLE MORRIS LASKER
United States District Court Judge,
Southern District,
New York, N. Y.

PAUL LIPSITT
Department of Psychiatry,
Harvard Medical School,
Boston, Mass.

Conference Participants

RICHARD T. LOUTTIT
Professor of Psychology,
Head, Department of Psychology
University of Massachusetts
Amherst, Mass.

RUDOLF MAGNONE
Regional Administrator for
*   Mental Retardation,*
Massachusetts Department of
*   Mental Health,*
West Springfield, Mass.

REPRESENTATIVE GARY MARBUT
National Association for
*   Retarded Children,*
Missoula, Mont.

JACK MARKER
Attorney,
National Institute of Mental Health,
Rockville, Md.

MERLE McCLUNG
Attorney,
Center for Law and Education
Harvard University,
Cambridge, Mass.

DAVID MECHANIC
Professor of Sociology,
University of Wisconsin,
Madison, Wis.

LEON NICKS
Psychology Consultant,
National Institute for Mental Health,
Boston, Mass.

MICHAEL PERLMAN
Regional Director of Legal Medicine,
Massachusetts Department of
*   Mental Health,*
West Springfield, Mass.

PAUL PIERCE
Patient-Inmate Advocate,
Maine Department of Mental Health and
*   Corrections,*
Augusta, Me.

JAY POMERANTZ
Regional Administrator for
*   Mental Health,*
Massachusetts Department of
*   Mental Health,*
West Springfield, Mass.

BENJAMIN RICCI
Chairman, Department of Exercise Science,
University of Massachusetts,
Amherst, Mass.

ELIZABETH SCHACK
Director of Children's Services,
Judicial Conference of the State of
*   New York,*
New York, N. Y.

SALEEM SHAH
Director,
Center for Studies of Crime and
*   Delinquency,*
National Institute of Mental Health,
Rockville, Md.

GOTTLIEB SIMON
Associate Administrative Officer
*   for Professional Affairs,*
American Psychological Association,
Washington, D. C.

STONEWALL STICKNEY
Former Commissioner of Alabama
*   Department of Mental Health,*
Montgomery, Ala.

Appendix B

CONFERENCE STAFF

Jeffrey Baker
Guillermo Bernal
William Fremouw
Avraham Frydman
Stuart Golann
Alexandra Kaplan

J. Gregory Olley
Janet Owens
Diana Scriver
Wendy Spence
Mrs. Richard J. Sturm
Castellano Turner

All of the University of Massachusetts, Amherst, Mass. Acknowledgment is gratefully made of the important contributions of the foregoing persons to the planning and accomplishment of the Conference and the preparation of the manuscript.

Index

PRODUCTION NOTE

This book has been set by Cemar Graphic Designs Ltd.
of Rockville Centre, New York,
in Primer and Helvetica typefaces.
Printing and binding were done at Noble Offset Printers,
of New York, New York.

Date Due

JUL 27 1981			
APR 3 0 1984			
MAY 2 1 1984			
APR 26 '96			
DEC 0 4 2009			